The Effects of
Drug
Regulation

The Effects of
Drug
Regulation

*A survey based on the European Studies
of Drug Regulation*

Graham Dukes

Regional Officer for Pharmaceuticals
and Drug Utilization
World Health Organization
Regional Office for Europe
Copenhagen
Denmark

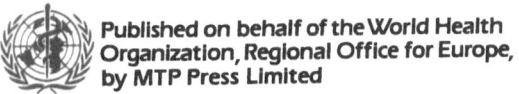
Published on behalf of the World Health
Organization, Regional Office for Europe,
by MTP Press Limited

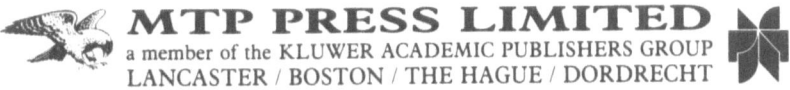
MTP PRESS LIMITED
a member of the KLUWER ACADEMIC PUBLISHERS GROUP
LANCASTER / BOSTON / THE HAGUE / DORDRECHT

The views expressed in this publication are those of the author and
an international group of experts and do not necessarily represent the decisions
or the stated policy of the World Health Organization.

Published in the UK and Europe by
MTP Press Limited
Falcon House
Lancaster, England

British Library Cataloguing in Publication Data

Dukes, Graham
    The effects of drug regulation
    1. Pharmaceutical policy
    I. Title
    363.1'946   RA401

ISBN-13: 978-94-011-7329-2   e-ISBN-13: 978-94-011-7327-8
DOI: 10.1007/978-94-011-7327-8

Published in the USA by
MTP Press
A division of Kluwer Boston Inc
190 Old Derby Street
Hingham, MA 02043, USA

Library of Congress Cataloging in Publication Data

Dukes, Graham.
    The effects of drug regulation

    Bibliography: p.
    Includes index
    1. Drugs—Law and legislation. 2. Drugs—Government
policy. I. Title. [DNLM: 1. Drugs—standards.
2. Drugs—Industry standards. 3. Legislation, Drug.
QV 771 D877e]
K3636.D85 1984   344'.04233   84–23394

ISBN-13: 978-94-011-7329-2

Contents

Acknowledgements

The writing of this book was only rendered possible by progress made with the European Studies of Drug Regulation since 1979. My thanks are due in the first place to my fellow members on the project team of the Studies; Inga Lunde carried out a great deal of the basic research and Almar Grimsson was instrumental in gaining the support of the Studies by the WHO Regional Office for Europe in 1980. The Studies themselves were only feasible because so much co-operation and help was provided by colleagues and friends in regulatory agencies, the pharmaceutical industry and academic centres.

A first draft of the text was discussed at a meeting held in Oslo in March 1984 made possible by generous support from the Health Services of Norway, and I am grateful to all the participants in that meeting for their many contributions to the text; a list of their names will be found in Annex 1. Finally, my thanks to Jill Turner for helping me to turn a committee document into a more readable text and to Sally Charnley and Liv Solem Andersen for their secretarial support.

Graham Dukes

Introduction

Most national governments have created agencies with the responsibility for deciding which medicinal drugs should be imported or manufactured and made available through their health systems. Many of these agencies were set up some twenty years ago in the wake of the thalidomide disaster. Since that time they have developed in quite different ways in response to national, cultural and economic influences. Their direct cost is very small in comparison to overall health budgets but their indirect effects, both in terms of health and the economy, can be substantial.

In 1980 the World Health Organization (WHO) Regional Office for Europe set up a series of studies of drug evaluation in the European region aimed at determining the effects of the work of regulatory agencies on the availability of drugs, on the pharmaceutical industry, and on the health of individuals in the countries concerned. This book sets that work in a historical context and describes the sources of the data used by the project team and the methods used by WHO and others in assessing the work of these agencies and its repercussions for the community. Finally, it presents an analysis of current knowledge and the plans and prospects for future research. The first draft of this book was presented to a meeting of experts in the field of drug regulation at Oslo in March 1984, and the present text embodies the views and conclusions of that meeting.

The assumption which underlies the creation of systems of

drug regulation is naturally that they will lead to better, safer and perhaps more economical medical treatment[9]. That assumption reflects in part the belief that if the pharmaceutical industry is allowed to function without any form of community control, it will not always act in society's best interests. Plainly pharmaceutical companies do vary a great deal as regards their technical standards, their scientific creativity and their social integrity. For that reason, because most or all manufacturers undoubtedly do sometimes make errors of judgement, and also because the industry is selling products the merits of which cannot easily be assessed by the individual prescriber or user, the view that some form of community control is needed is today hardly disputed. To say that, however, is not to justify every existing form of regulation, and to point to some of the weaknesses in the pharmaceutical industry is not to condemn all that is valuable in that industry.

Assumptions and hypotheses about health legislation and regulation, like those in any area of medicine, need to be reassessed critically as knowledge and experience increase; there must be no automatism and no thoughtless growth of restriction. Writing on legal principles of public health administration as long ago as 1914, Wigmore said:

'It is modern science that has vastly enlarged the scope of modern law. We have found that the scope of measures necessary for common defense calls for this enlargement of function. The law has become involved in the necessities of applied science. Is it yet equal to the task? Will old and settled principles serve? Do the new measures call merely for new applications of old principles, or for their destruction and the creation of new ones? Is it merely a changed phase of the conflict between individual liberty and general welfare – between executive discretion and fixed law, – between officialism and laissez faire?'[1]

Despite such sentiments, only sporadic attempts have been made to determine the effect of legal regulation in the field of

health, and even at the present day they are looked on as
novel. As recently as November 1983, in the *Journal of the
American Medical Association,* Lundberg recalled that:

'Some years ago, I was consulted by a state employee in
California regarding a proposed new laboratory regulation. I
asked him what the effect of a particular earlier regulation
had been. He said he didn't know and that there had been no
study of it. I asked why they were proposing a new regulation when they did not know the effect of the older one.
Recently, when discussing the quality assurance programs
that highlight current policy of the Joint Commission on
Accreditation of Hospitals, I asked what scientific evidence
there was that documented a change in quality produced by
these elaborate new standards. I was told there had been no
such studies and no data existed to answer the question . . .'[17]

The drama of thalidomide in 1961 may have justified the rapid
passage of new drug legislation twenty years ago, but it does
not necessarily justify enacting or maintaining exactly the same
legislation today. Since that time, so much experience, both
favourable and unfavourable, has been gained in drawing up,
applying and amending drug laws and regulations that one can
and must learn from it. There has fortunately been no repeti-
tion of the thalidomide disaster, but other misadventures
involving new drugs have occurred and some of them have
affected many more individuals than did thalidomide. Most of
these events have provided some indication as to how such
problems might be avoided in the future, and why existing
regulations failed to prevent them. During this same period,
too, changes have taken place in the drug industry, some no
doubt spontaneous, some apparently fostered by the development of comprehensive legislation; the industry of 1984 may
need to be regulated in a manner different from the industry as
it existed in 1961.

If over-regulation, under-regulation or inappropriate regulation are to be avoided, the effects of any form of health

regulation need to be kept constantly under review. That principle, which has become increasingly recognized by the World Health Organization, applies to all those health fields (including matters as diverse as environmental protection, workers' health and medical education) in which society finds it necessary to set and enforce standards. It is not always easy, however, to determine to what extent legislative or regulatory measures have turned out to be effective. Just as when testing a new drug, one should ideally study the effects of a new law under controlled conditions; means of doing this have been developed in several fields (e.g. chemical safety, automobile safety) and the drug field provides a compact and important area in which such techniques can be further developed, and the findings quickly put to good use[55].

1

The background

1. THE ORIGINS OF DRUG REGULATION

In one form or another, a degree of community control on medicines and medicinal therapy is very old. Penn[2] has cited examples from ancient Egypt and the Old Testament; in mediaeval Moslem countries, an official health inspector, the *muhtasib*, was charged with ensuring that apothecaries maintained sufficient standards:

> '. . . it is necessary that the muhtasib make them fearful, try them and warn them against imprisonment. He must caution them with punishment. Their syrups and drugs may be inspected at any time after their shops are closed for the night . . .'[3]

With the apothecary or retail pharmacist responsible throughout a great part of history not only for selling drugs but also for preparing them, legislation was concerned largely with his professional standards. In England in 1540, the College of Physicians was given the right to search apothecaries' shops for drugs that were:

> . . . defective, corrupted and not meet nor convenient to be ministered in any medicine for the health of mans body . . .'[4]

Concern with the commercial production of drugs and with the nascent pharmaceutical industry first became evident in the seventeenth century. The Great Plague of London in 1665 occurred at a time when printing and the establishment of the newspaper press had rendered it feasible and attractive to advertise wares, including medicines, to the public, leading to production on a larger scale[5]. As Daniel Defoe wrote, reconstructing the scene many years later:

> 'It is incredible and scarce to be imagined how the Posts of Houses and the Corners of Streets were plastered over with Doctor's Bills and Papers of Ignorant Fellows. Quacking and tampering with Physick, and inviting the People to come to them for Remedies; which was generally set off with such flourisches as these, viz., Infallible preventative Pills against the Plague, Never-Failing Preservatives against the Infection, Sovereign Cordials against the Corruption of the Air . . .'[132]

The tradition of drug advertising, good or bad, established at that period continued and developed throughout the eighteenth century. The vogue for inorganic metallic remedies, including highly noxious compounds based on arsenic and mercury, which grew up at that time was very largely fostered by public advertising. Not surprisingly, in 1799 a contributor to a medical journal proposed to the legislature:

> '. . . the propriety of erecting a public board composed of the most eminent physicians for the examination, analyzation and approbation of every medicine before an advertisement should be admitted into any newspaper or any other periodical publication and before it should be vended in any manner whatsoever . . .'[6]

Most of the drug legislation passed during the century which followed nevertheless still dealt only with the training of pharmacists, the establishment of pharmacies, and to some extent the role of the pharmaceutical profession in ensuring adequate quality standards for drugs. The first official lists of drugs had been introduced in the sixteenth century when cities in Italy and Germany published pharmacopoeias which were intended to guide the formulation and the quality of drugs; by the nineteenth century pharmacopoeias had achieved legal or quasilegal status in most European countries. Concepts of efficacy and safety did not however feature in the pharmacopoeias, nor did they find their way into the law; there was indeed no reason why they should do so, except for the purpose of countering frank charlatanism, so long as most medicines in use were derived from herbs, the properties of which were thought to have been sufficiently well defined by long experience.

During the nineteenth century, however, pressure for further change did emerge. It came largely from independent investigators and protest movements, as a reaction to the growth of the 'patient medicine' industry which followed the industrial revolution and the rise of a large urban working class[5]. While among the medicines made for the masses there were innocent herbal laxatives, sedatives, expectorants and antacids which were sold as such, intensive advertising was also conducted for what were claimed to be remedies for tuberculosis, cancer and syphilis. Typical of the demands for reform were those advanced by the Bruinsma brothers in the Netherlands in a book published in 1878, presenting an analysis of many of the useless remedies on sale, the methods used to sell them, and the true cost of their ingredients[7]. In due course, a certain number of countries indeed did pass ordinances at least prohibiting the public advertising of drugs for the cure of contagious and malignant diseases.

In the meantime, the development of chemical synthetic techniques began to produce a new generation of potent remedies, typified by the organic arsenical arsphenamine (Ehrlich, 1907). Pharmacists, who willingly accepted legal responsibility for drugs which they had compounded themselves, soon began to question the extent of their responsibilities for these entirely new drugs manufactured on a large scale by the chemical industry. A long time passed, however, before a series of misadventures began to underline the need for some form of community control on new drug products. Even in the United States it was not until 1937 that the Elixir of Sulfonamide tragedy (involving the untested use of diethylene glycol as a solvent for sulfanilamide, resulting in numerous fatalities) triggered the establishment of an administrative procedure for the premarketing clearance of products of uncertain safety[8].

Various attempts to reduce risk were made in Europe during the interwar period. Some countries set up limited systems of drug registration, factory inspectorates or control laboratories; the regulations upon which these were based were however often very general in nature and similar to those in force for foodstuffs at the time; some of the new systems of registration, insofar as they existed, involved purely administrative formalities. Here and there official or voluntary controls on advertising and prescription were introduced. A very few countries, such as the United States, also tackled the problem of deceptive labelling, i.e. the entire question of the claims made for a drug[37]. In addition, of course, most countries had special narcotics regulations intended to fulfil their obligations under international conventions[9]. In other respects, even by the middle of the twentieth century, the efficacy and safety of new drugs had still scarcely become community concerns.

By that time, however, the rapid expansion in the number of synthetic drugs had greatly increased the chances not only of achieving therapeutic advances but also of creating new risks. In the latter respect, the turning point may be said to have come on November 18th 1961 when the pediatrician Dr Widukind Lenz informed a group of physicians meeting in Düsseldorf that he had tentatively traced a current outbreak of phocomelia, involving gross foetal deformities, to the use in pregnancy of the new hypnotic drug thalidomide[10]. The drug, which already proved neurotoxic, was withdrawn shortly afterwards; the realization of the injury which it had caused provided the greatest single impulse to the development of new drug legislation in Europe and elsewhere. It also provided important precedents as regards the responsibility of manufacturers at civil law (tort) for the consequences of injury caused by their products; tort liability was subsequently to become an important factor influencing the behaviour of many pharmaceutical companies.

Even after the thalidomide disaster, the extent of which was limited only by the fact that the drug had been marketed only in a few countries, the introduction of preventative legislation was largely directed to safety issues and not to efficacy, though the Kefauver amendments to United States drug law in 1962 were concerned with both efficacy and safety. Only a very few countries, notably Norway and Sweden, where the relevant legislation dated from 1928 and 1935 respectively, had gained experience with systems to assess the efficacy of new drugs[12]. Writing as late as 1967 on behalf of the then (British) Committee on Safety of Drugs, a body constituted on a voluntary basis but with official collaboration and approval, Dunlop stressed that: 'The Committee's remit does not impose upon it any responsibility to consider the efficacy of drugs except in so far as their safety is concerned. Therefore, the Committee's clearance of a drug for marketing does not necessarily imply their approval of it as a remedy . . .'[11]

The introduction of reasonable proof of efficacy as a basic element in drug regulation did not become at all generally accepted until the growth of clinical pharmacology during the 1960s and 1970s both demonstrated the inadequacy of existing evidence and provided the tools with which to determine whether a drug was truly effective in man or not. Furthermore concepts such as the use of controlled clinical trials were slow to cross national boundaries.

Forces moulding the regulatory pattern   The few examples given here remind us that the introduction of regulation in the drug field has often occurred as a response to disasters; the response has generally been slow and often forthcoming only after a great deal of pressure has been exerted at the political level. The pharmaceutical industry has tended to oppose these pressures, arguing the case for self-regulation[122], occasionally in very absolute terms. As Wells[85], writing on behalf of the British pharmaceutical industry, argues: 'The implied assumption of the regulatory protagonists that intervention via statutory measures is necessary to ensure adequate testing of new medicines is . . . questionable. It fails to recognize that the pharmaceutical industry's credibility and hence livelihood is founded on the manufacture of only safe, efficacious and high quality medicines'.

Others have questioned the doctrine of self-regulation, particularly in view of the fact that the newly established agencies found so many things in need of correction. When in the United Kingdom in 1971 the Medicines Act (1968) was implemented over 3600 companies registered their already marketed products under some 39,000 product licences of right; of these by 1983 some 22,000 had been withdrawn from the market[156]. Griffin[168] has adduced this as persuasive evidence of the inadequacy of voluntary regulation in certain respects, though it obviously can and must complement any form of official regulation. Similar conclusions have been attached by Laporte[169] to the marked decline in the number of products in Spain following the introduction of more effective regulatory mechanisms (Table I)[157].

Table I Pharmaceutical presentations and specialities on sale in Spain

PRESENTATIONS	SPECIALITIES
1977 – 18,000*	1977 – 10,000*
1978 – 16,500*	1978 – 9,200*
1983 – 14,500	1983 – 8,000

*In these years, OTC products in Spain (i.e. self-medication products sold over the counter) were negligible in number. These figures refer only to 'ethicals' i.e. products primarily intended for use under a physician's supervision.

It is striking that the debate on drug regulation has been conducted largely at the political and industrial level, with more recent participation from the consumer movement. A far less prominent role in the debate has been played by the professions, though medical associations have sometimes expressed concern about measures which might limit the physician's freedom of choice in prescribing.

It is also striking that these discussions on drug regulation have been conducted largely on matters of principle, with emotional arguments playing a major role in enlisting support. Insofar as the debate has been documented, one often finds that the evidence presented has been fragmentary or selected to suit the cause of special pleading on one side or the other. Cause and effect relationships have remained unproved if only because many of the essential data on risks and effective means of avoiding them have not been available. It has therefore not been easy for policy makers to form an objective view of the regulations needed by society; their decisions may have been determined largely by the various pressures brought to bear on them.

This book is not intended to provide a full account of the controversy, but it has to be summarized later in this Chapter since the arguments advanced for and against drug regulation point to many of the elements which need to be examined if we are to determine whether regulation has indeed lived up to the high expectations of some or the worst expectations of others.

Differences and similarities in national regulatory development Because of varying national situations and the differing pressures exerted on policy makers, it is not surprising that drug legislation and regulation developed in quite different ways in different countries. Even between countries with relatively similar traditions, there can be marked differences in regulatory policies. Analysing the Nordic situation in 1983, Granat *et al.*[64] noted that the number of products marketed ranged from 1,164 in Iceland (728 brand names) to 3,824 in Denmark (2,201 brand names); the acceptance rate on drugs of international significance ranged over a four-year period from 40% in Norway to 78% in Finland.

If one looks at a broader area of Europe, much greater divergences in drug policy between countries emerge, as reflected for example in estimates of the total number of marketed products or the number of preparations listed in the physician's compendium (Tables II and III). In a five-country comparison over the period 1960–1981[78] Hass *et al.* found that of the new molecules introduced in one or more of these countries 60–70% were marketed in France, the Federal Republic of Germany and Italy but only 46% in the United Kingdom and about 32% (after some delay) in the United States.

Some such variations from one major country to another

Table II Estimated numbers of specialities on some European markets 1977/1978[57]

Federal Republic of Germany	120,000	(15,000)
United Kingdom	26,000	(15,000)
Italy	13,700	
Belgium	7,900	
France	7,800	
Ireland	7,400	
Luxemburg	7,300	
Finland	3,700	
Netherlands	3,400	
Sweden	2,700	
Norway	1,870	
Iceland	1,180	

These figures were based on data supplied by members of the staff of the regulatory agencies. However, the higher figures cited for the United Kingdom and the Federal Republic of Germany include many products which only marginally qualify as specialities, especially homeopathic drugs and drugs which are prepared and sold only in a single pharmacy (and in the case of the Federal Republic of Germany, herbal teas); the lower figures provide a better basis for comparison. Products licensed as medical products in some countries are excluded in others. The figures represent a period before the influence of harmonization of drug laws could have been felt. They exclude sera, vaccines and (in the case of European Community member states) veterinary drugs but they do include all the various dosage strengths and forms of each product.

Table III Numbers of drugs listed in physicians' compendia 1981

Country	Source	Active substances	Products	Formulations
France	Vidal	1,000	2,300	4,000
Germany,				
Fed. Rep. of	Rote Liste	2,550	8,900	11,155
Sweden	FASS	750	1,600	2,500
UK	MIMS	1,100	2,100	3,900
USA	P.D.R.	1,200	6,000	12,000

These figures were supplied to the project team of the European Studies of Drug Regulation in 1981 by the International Federation of Pharmaceutical Manufacturers' Associations. In some countries the compendia omit many drugs intended for use by specialists such as ear, nose and throat preparations and contrast media.

extend even to matters on which one might reasonably expect a scientific consensus, such as the list of approved indications for a well-studied drug like cimetidine, already available for a number of years[52]. Certain of these divergent decisions on an individual drug naturally reflect the subjective element in therapeutic judgements, further influenced by the environment in which they are exercised. More consistent differences in national regulatory tradition may to some extent even be medically defensible. As Quantock has put it, speaking from the side of the pharmaceutical industry: 'Different countries have their own special problems. Ethnic differences lead to dosage variations. Varying health care standards require different therapeutic approaches, and local therapeutic traditions have developed over the centuries and bring their own complexities.'[36] What that in practice seems to mean is that a regulatory authority may sometimes find itself obliged to go along with national medical practice and opinion irrespective of what pure scientific judgement may dictate.

   Where differences in regulatory tradition go beyond what one would expect on medical grounds they may also reflect economic and structural divergences. A country with little or no innovative industry and a tradition of centralization may be more prone to enact restrictive laws – in what it sees as the public health interest – than will a more permissive country with a major innovative and exporting industry. In certain cases (for example in the field of contraceptives and abortifacients) standards adopted may reflect religious or ethical norms in a particular region[19].

The broadest difference in drug regulatory policies, however, ranging from general restrictiveness at one extreme to general permissiveness at the other, is that between the southern and the northern parts of Europe; it seems to reflect quite basic variations in cultural tradition[57] which are equally reflected in the doctor's prescribing habits and the public's expectations. The demand for drugs between northern and southern Europe differs not only when one looks at the numbers of drugs marketed but also at the turnover of the pharmaceutical industry, drug utilization statistics, and the numbers of items likely to be dispensed on a single prescription. One can also compare the proportion of the population's income spent on drugs in various countries. In 1975 this was found to be 0.82% for England and Wales, 1.41% for Belgium, 1.70% for France and 2.15% for Italy[66], though of course these figures are also influenced by economic factors. Very similar figures have been produced more recently by Griffiths[125].

One can also find plenty of variations in specific types of demand from one part of Europe to another. As Klaes *et al.*[66] put it:

'In Germany cardiac insufficiency plays a major role in medicine. Medicines corresponding to this are prescribed very much more frequently than in other countries. Hypotension is regarded in Germany as a disease; elsewhere it is only considered to be pathological when it is very severe. In France, hepatic disorders receive a great deal of attention, in Great Britain respiratory disorders. As far as the nature of drug products is concerned: the so-called fixed combinations are popular in therapy in Germany. The situation is quite different in Britain where mono-preparations (with one active component) are of relatively greater importance. This degree of differentiation can go so far that in many countries (e.g. Denmark) fixed combinations are as a matter of principle not allowed to be sold with a few exceptions. Although such differences have not been systematically investigated, their potential importance must be stressed.'

Klaes' observations as regards fixed combinations can be readily confirmed from other sources. What is publicly known of discussions on new drug applications within the European Community's expert committees shows, for example, that the resistance to fixed combinations in Denmark is still virtually absolute.

Other studies have looked in some depth at national divergences as regards individual therapeutic groups. In a European study of the regulation of drugs for treatment or prevention of senile dementia, which noted strikingly different practices from country to country, it was pointed out that 'there is clearly a widespread and insatiable demand from physicians and from the public for drugs which at least appear to provide some hope of relief for the cerebral disorders of the aged. The extent to which a government agency can acquiesce to such a demand even where it entails approving (or at least continuing to tolerate) the sale of preparations of dubious value is a matter of national mentality; one nation is more paternalistic towards its physicians and its public in such matters than another.'[67]

Differences such as these are not mere vestiges of abandoned policies; regulatory agencies still appear to be strongly influenced by national factors. In one of his later studies Hass[112] used an ingenious technique to compare the current availability of the world's 100 top-selling drugs in eleven countries, limiting his study to drugs first introduced on the world market in 1963 or later. The number of these actually on sale in the individual countries ranged from 50 in Norway to 92 in Italy. When he broke down these figures according to the types of drugs available he found marked differences in national spectra. There was a very close similarity in the

spectrum between France and Italy and a progressively declining degree of correspondence as one compared Italy to the
Federal Republic of Germany, the Federal Republic of Germany to Switzerland and Switzerland to the United Kingdom.
A second cluster of similar countries with respect to the
spectrum of drugs sold comprised Canada, Australia and the
United States. A third and distinctly different cluster comprised Norway and Sweden.

One might advance the hypothesis that regulatory and
marketing patterns do not merely follow national traditions but
also help to fortify and perpetuate them. Whether or not that is
in the public interest – for example as regards the widespread
use of digitalis preparations on the middle aged in the Federal
Republic of Germany – is obviously a matter which needs to be
studied in detail. It is almost inconceivable that the medicinal
needs of the population in the ten member states of the
European Community really differ so greatly as the differences
in their current drug markets would suggest.

International trends and experience   The differences, often
very wide, between regulatory requirements and practices in
different countries have always been a source of concern to the
pharmaceutical industry, particularly because of the time and
expense involved in preparing numerous divergent new drug
applications for a single product, which often necessitate
repeating scientific work[20]. The introduction of a uniform
requirement as regards both the content and form of scientific
data would greatly simplify matters; it should also be feasible,
for the scientific investigations required are usually broadly
similar. At one time, the drug industry was for such reasons a
prominent advocate of the adoption of international standards.
It is interesting to recall that, had that view become generally
accepted, a firm legal basis for the adoption of worldwide
standards could have been found in Articles 2 and 21 of the
World Health Organization's constitution (cited by
Fatturusso[170]). It is not easy to discover exactly why the
pharmaceutical industry subsequently became much more hesi-

tant on the issue, but some factors are quite clear. For one thing, it is widely realized that national traditions in the interpretation of written rules differ greatly; whereas one type of administration will take them only as a starting point for individual decisions based on common sense and sound judgement, others will be prone to apply them literally and rigidly under all circumstances. Another factor which may well have changed industry's approach was the experience with the only supranational drug registration system ever to have been put into operation, one which was operative in the three Benelux countries from 1973 to 1978. There is no doubt that in some cases an individual country did withdraw its objections to a product in the light of arguments from the other member states; by and large, however, there seems to have been a trend in Benelux to adopt the most restrictive norms pertaining in any of the three countries[21]. It was perhaps this venture, more than anything else, which caused the pharmaceutical industry to argue from that time onwards for 'mutual recognition' of regulatory decisions, particularly in the European Community[115].

The principal current developments leading to a greater measure of regulatory uniformity in certain groups of countries may be summarized here as follows.

The influence of pharmacopoeias These played a role in creating uniform norms long before the era of modern drug regulation, particularly because major national pharmacopoeias were followed outside their own frontiers; in more recent years, common pharmacopoeias (notably the Nordic, European and International Pharmacopoeia) have extended this role.

The European Community Arrangements were introduced in 1976 which encouraged manufacturers to make a single application to the Committee for Proprietary Medicinal Products, part of the European Communities Commission, and this scheme has been moderately successful[152]. As early as 1979, however, it had become clear that, with divergences in regulatory practice as extreme as those which existed in the Community, mutual recognition of (positive) regulatory decisions would be unacceptable to the various member states, since it would have undermined systems which, at the national level, were conceived as being essential to the maintenance of public health[22]; since 1983 the ultimate aim of the Commission has been mutual recognition, but this aim is not included in the latest amendments to the Directives[162]. What is important is that a common pattern of legislation and common guidelines have been adopted throughout the Community.

The Council for Mutual Economic Assistance (CMEA)   The Member States of CMEA are collaborating to develop recommended uniform standards for pre-clinical, clinical-pharmacological and clinical investigation of new drugs. As in the European Community, guidelines have been issued for this purpose.

Nordic collaboration   The Nordic countries have for some decades aimed at harmonizing their regulatory practices. Initially this was mainly in the field of drug standardization and resulted in the compilation and publication of the Nordic Pharmacopoeia in 1963. The parliamentary assembly of the Nordic Council set up a working group in the early sixties to make recommendations for a formalized cooperation between the five countries in the field of drug assessment and registration. The report (1969) of this working group recommended as principal steps the establishment of a convention for Nordic drug registration, the creation of a drug research fund and the setting up of a Nordic Council on Medicines. The implementation of the first two recommendations was postponed but the Nordic Council on Medicines was formally established in 1975 with a broad mandate to work towards harmonization of legislation and administrative practices in the Nordic countries. The Council has carried out a number of harmonization activities, the most important ones being the elaboration of common Nordic guidelines for clinical trials, drug applications and Nordic Statistics on Medicines which includes classification and methodology for drug utilization studies.

European Free Trade Area The EFTA has made arrangements for the mutual exchange of evaluation protocols between its regulatory agencies on request, and for mutual recognition of inspection.

Informal contacts Various informal meetings of regulatory agencies having similar philosophies are held regularly to discuss common problems and approaches.

Activities of the World Health Organization The many activities of WHO in this field have included the organization of both global meetings of regulatory agencies (since 1980) and European regional meetings (annually since 1972). These play an important role in elucidating common principles and establishing contacts between regulatory officials which often continue on an informal basis between meetings.

As a result of such developments, differences in regulatory tradition have certainly declined to some extent. If one might venture a guess as to the single most important influence leading to harmonization then it is not any complex regional or global system but the establishment of personal and informal contacts between regulators across frontiers. Informal consultation is now common throughout Europe before national decisions are taken on important issues. The effects of these developments may not be quantifiable but they are quite clearly there. It may be that these unofficial and unrecognized activities will continue to provide the only substantial contribution to harmonization until real progress has been made towards finding an objective approach to drug regulation which can be applied globally.

The present and potential scope of drug regulation   It is often said that regulation is intended to ensure that medicines will, so far as possible, be well made, efficacious and safe. In some countries, however, regulation goes much further (Table IV); the extent to which these other matters are officially regulated from country to country shows marked differences in what Klaes *et al.* call the 'intensity' or 'density' of drug regulation. The pharmaceutical industry and market are also affected by more general forms of regulation, such as those concerned with monopolies, patent protection, workers' health and the environment. Any of these may be just as influential as regulations specific to medicines. Finally, some drug regulatory agencies have authority to play a more active medical role, for

Table IV   Matters subject to regulation in certain countries

---

Development and investigation
    Animal studies (scientific and ethical aspects)
    Safety and comparative safety in man
    Efficacy and comparative efficacy in man
    Clinical trials (protocols, licensing of investigators)
    Efficacy/safety ratio
    Adverse reaction monitoring

Manufacture
    Manufacturing conditions
    Quality (and quality control procedures); stability
    Packaging (adequacy, childproof closure, labelling)

Marketing
    Data sheet and directions folder (indications, warning, dosage etc.)
    Advertising (Written, oral); sampling and other inducements to
        prescribe
    Distribution
    Classes of physicians permitted to prescribe a certain drug
    Prescription requirements
    Eligibility for health service payment
    Pricing
    Products for export

---

example in distributing information to doctors. The effects of such activities, too, may need to be evaluated.

2. THE REGULATORY CONTROVERSY

For those working in the pharmaceutical field the controversy about drug regulation may seem to be unique. In fact it is only one facet of a much broader controversy around social regulation in general[174]. Martin[76] has summarized the history of what he calls 'the contemporary controversy over the compatibility between the expansion of social regulation in recent years and the restoration of economic growth and employment'. He goes on:

'Reflecting the successful political expression of rapidly burgeoning concern over the safety and quality of working conditions, the environment, and products, social standards of production began to be established on a larger scale in many of the advanced societies during the 1970s. While the policies through which this has been done have been uneven in their effectiveness they have undoubtedly contributed to some improvement in the quality of life and arrested some of the deterioration that was becoming an increasingly apparent byproduct of uncontrolled growth. Late as it was in the long postwar period of growth, then, public policy was increasingly extended from concern with the rate and stability of growth to previously neglected aspects of its composition. As the crisis plaguing the international economy since the middle of the last decade persisted, however, resistance to social regulation intensified. Particularly in the United States, such regulation has been charged with imposing costly burdens on the economy, fueling inflation, impairing the international competitiveness of firms, and jeopardizing their employees' jobs. This is, indeed, the rationale for the current wave of "regulatory relief" in the U.S. that has almost halted the extension of social regulation and significantly eroded existing standards as well as the agencies for implementing them. While social regulation, in its somewhat different forms, has evidently not been attacked to the same degree in Western Europe, there too, economic stagnation has lent plausibility to the view that workplace, environment and product standards impose economic costs which are an obstacle to the restoration of growth and employment . . .'[76].

In the pharmacueticals field this controversy has been conducted at varying levels of sophistication. As Crout has written[110]:

'There is a positive side to this debate about regulation which has been highly beneficial – that is, it has served to highlight to the public how regulators conduct their business. There is also a growing understanding of the complexity of regulatory decisions. Those with simple solutions are being challenged to think more broadly. On the negative side, however, there is a thoughtless, almost reflex lashing out against regulation in some circles that is disturbing. While emotional outbursts against the bureaucracy or the government in general are useful in highlighting a problem, they are usually not helpful in articulating a solution to that problem . . .'

An example of an emotionally loaded statement being used to recruit support is the familiar argument that 'some regulatory agencies are now requiring such concentration on safety that the benefits to patients are actually being jeopardized' (quoted by Cromie[24]). The argument is not necessarily wrong; certainly there are circumstances in which regulatory delay could deprive patients of a life-saving drug. But such an argument, advanced in Europe, needs to be backed up by concrete European examples. There is a strong tendency to extrapolate from the most cautious acts of the United States Federal Food and Drug Administration to the policies of European agencies, most of which are very different. Even the situation in the United States has sometimes been interpreted in a curious manner. One much quoted statement, dating from

1977, is to the effect that 'the eleven years of delay in introducing beta-blockers into the United States for indications other than arrythmias, killed a quarter of a million Americans'[25]; it was this which led Cromie to speak of the 'mass murder activities of regulatory authorities'[24] and which is still being cited in documents in which one would hope to find a scientific view of drug control problems[122]. The unapproved indications in question were in fact angina pectoris and hypertension; for both, alternative forms of medication were available with comparable life-saving potential, a fact which was not taken into account when the estimate of a quarter of a million deaths was made; in actual fact, too, the delay in approval for angina pectoris was only six years, and prior to approval the beta-blocker propranolol (already available for arrhythmias) appears to have been widely used for both angina and hypertension.

Figures presented on the situation in Europe are again sometimes very misleading or frankly incorrect. Cromie, again, writing in 1978 on 'the average duration of tests required by the Committee on Safety of Medicines for a chronically adminis- tered medicine'[24] estimated this as having been 5.4 years in 1965, 10.0 years in 1971 and 17.6 years at the time of writing; he added that 'at this rate the medicines available in the year 2000 would need about 100 years of work before Product Licence submission'. The graphic presentation on which this extrapolation is based reflects however the assumption that the biological work (some 12 years) and the clinical work (5 years) will be conducted consecutively rather than in parallel; the figures cited are also much in excess of what the Committee at that time required. Finally, the estimates are strongly influ- enced by the growing complexity of the chemical and phar- maceutical work involved in developing a new drug, a change which is due to scientific rather than regulatory changes.

These few citations are not intended to throw any unfavour- able light either on the underlying arguments or on the authors involved; they merely serve to illustrate the fact that even good arguments for or against drug regulation have sometimes been backed by poor or invalid evidence; anyone claiming at the present day to produce usable data on the effects of regulation must contrive to do a great deal better.

Pressures to revise and relax regulation Much of the argument against what is considered to be excessive regulation has been put forward by the pharmaceutical industry. Sometimes it has argued the case openly in its own economic interest, sometimes it has pointed to risks which regulation may create for the prescriber or his patient. To a degree, indeed, it has sought to mobilize opinion in the medical profession, pressing the view that the physician's freedom to prescribe is endangered by regulatory trends. Typical of this was the fact that a meeting organized in London by pharmaceutical industry staff in 1979 under the title 'Risk and regulation in medicine' was later published with the added sub-title: 'the fettered physician'[32].

The main case advanced by the pharmaceutical industry rests however on three inter-related arguments, all three of which need to be taken seriously.

The first is the *public health risk*, i.e. the danger that excessive regulation will not only delay the marketing of useful new drugs currently emerging from research and development but will also basically hinder the research process and dam the flow of useful new products. Writing in 1978, Cromie anticipated a 'barren harvest brought about by the regulatory requirements' of the preceding decade[24]; others have contested this view[56]. The argument has been pressed particularly strongly as regards what are said to be excessive demands for toxicity testing[104], although until recently specific examples were very rarely presented.

Secondly, much is made of the *industrial risk*, i.e. that the return on investment will decline to a point where the pharmaceutical industry will no longer attract sufficient capital to survive or will move into other and more attractive manufacturing fields. A particular argument has been that the period taken to develop, register and market a new drug will approach or even exceed the period of patent protection[91]. Similar views have been presented on pricing policies; the president of the Italian industry association has been quoted as declaring that his government 'was to blame for the erosion of the national pharmaceutical industry and risked killing it off entirely'[171].

Thirdly, there is said to be a *national economic risk*, i.e. a danger that adverse effects on the drug industry will harm national interests by causing unemployment and decreasing export earnings, particularly when firms operating in a heavily regulated environment find themselves unable to compete on world markets with freer foreign undertakings.

Pressures to intensify regulation   By contrast, pressures to intensify and extend regulatory mechanisms are recognizable in most countries – even in Scandinavia where the existing stringent policies are still considered by some to provide insufficient protection[138]. These pressures have emanated largely from four interrelated sources:

Drug disasters (see above). Thalidomide is the classic example of a drug disaster, but there continue to be others, and they may have been more directly influential than a scientific consensus in influencing regulation. In 1980, for example, a WHO symposium noted a broad consensus of opinion that drugs likely to be used in the elderly should first be tested in the elderly[14]. The immediate stimulus to the subsequent introduction of requirements to this effect in various countries was however widely regarded as the series of fatalities produced by benoxaprofen in the elderly in 1982[16]. To be fair, however, some bodies, such as the United Kingdom's Committee on Safety of Medicines, had indeed taken action to draft such requirements before the first reports of benoxaprofen toxicity were received[15].

The importance of adverse reactions in influencing policy decisions seems to depend not only upon their severity and percentage incidence but also upon the absolute number of reactions reported. Even where the percentage incidence is extremely low the fact that the drug in question is widely sold and the total number of complications is thus considerable renders the effect 'visible' in the public mind and makes it a matter of sufficient public health importance to require action.

Public pressure can be exerted independently of any specific disaster or other event. Consumer organizations (and others who consider that they are acting in the consumer's interest) have been active in urging public authorities to impose additional or more rigid restrictions on the drug market; some, such as Health Action International, are dedicated largely to this purpose[18]. The mass media have often taken a similar view, criticizing existing regulatory bodies for laxity[89, 123, 124]. Some of these views have been inspired by acute drug disasters, others by the exposure of more chronic problems, e.g. those relating to the safety of phenylbutazone and oxyphenbutazone, which came to a head largely as a result of pressures from action groups in the United States and Sweden late in 1983[23, 148]. Although one might also expect some part of the public to call for faster and simpler introduction of new drugs, this has hardly happened outside the United States where the concept of the 'drug lag', originally presented by Lasagna and further developed by Wardell[77], has been very heavily publicized[38, 39, 40]. Even in the United States, however, agencies are more likely to be criticized in the mass media for failure to prevent injury than for excessive stringency. As Cromie has said: 'Regulatory authorities . . . are unlikely to receive much public plaudit for speeding new medicines through the regulatory process, but they will certainly be blamed if a foreseeable or even an unforseeable hazard was missed . . .'[24].

Most regulatory agencies have now and again given in to acute public pressure, generally catalyzed by the media, and taken precipitous (generally negative) decisions on drugs. Wade[33] has recalled how, after the premature disclosure in 1970 of the preliminary results of the still disputed University Group Diabetes Programme study of oral antidiabetic drugs a newspaper columnist in the United States wrote (of tolbutamide) that 'the study suggests . . . that at least 8,000 users of the drug die prematurely every year in the United States alone'. Shortly afterwards – in what was widely seen as a direct consequence of such newspaper statements – a warning as to the hazards of all sulfonylurea drugs was issued by the Food and Drug Administration (FDA). Sometimes a sudden upsurge of public concern seems to have been due to a deliberate leak from a drug regulatory agency, so creating a climate of opinion favourable to the announcement of its decision.

The *medical profession* can be seen as a third source of pressure. Although, as already pointed out, practitioners generally have not been very active in the regulatory debate, some medical editors have expressed concern at possible over-regulation[139, 140]. Physicians and pharmacologists have sometimes debated the issue of regulation versus innovation at scientific meetings without finding original solutions[141]. Clinical pharmacologists have been more prone to point to failings in current systems for protecting the public interest; certain of them have suggested the need for regulatory or other restraints on the over-exuberant marketing of new products, which in several instances has led to an unnecessarily high incidence of serious adverse effects not recognized prior to marketing[172]. Offerhaus, discussing several such instances, suggests that 'Either the barriers to be surmounted before registration must be set higher, or the possibility of imposing conditions on marketing licences must be created or extended'[70].

Finally there is the role of *political pressure*. The idea that society should exert more rigid control on a large and multinational industry has been advanced actively from those political groupings advocating this approach to industry in general[134]. Some political pressure has naturally gone in the opposite direction, with allegations that agencies are stifling a productive industry; this has happened most markedly in the United States because of evidence of the so-called 'drug lag' in that country as documented by the General Accounting Office report[79] and by Wardell's group[73]. Even there, however, political pressure to intensify regulation has been intense. As a former Commissioner of the FDA remarked as long ago as

1974: '. . . in all of FDA's history I am unable to find a single instance where a Congressional committee investigated the *failure* of FDA to approve a new drug. But the times when hearings have been held to criticize our approval of new drugs have been so frequent that we aren't able to count them . . .'[95]. Similar pressures can be noted in debates in the United Kingdom Parliament, following the withdrawal of benoxaprofen[123] and in other European legislatures.

One might add to this list of overt or hidden pressures tending to result in more stringent regulation the very natural tendency of a professional drug regulator, in cases of doubt, to take the course safest for himself, which is often the most restrictive one. The danger that this will happen may well be greater in a country where an individual assessor bears the brunt of the responsibility for an official decision, than in those many European countries where decisions are taken by (or on the advice of) a committee of experts.

Development of the controversy If one looks back at the regulatory controversy over the last decade, one can see how the debate in most countries has oscillated, often from one extreme to the other, depending on events. In the years immediately following the thalidomide disaster, public and political opinion was overwhelmingly in favour of far more stringent regulatory control. Early in the 1970's after another decade had gone by without major drug dramas, voices suggesting the need to relax regulation were increasingly heard. In 1974 renewed questioning as to the adequacy of regulatory demands followed the practolol incident. Thereafter a new wave of protest against regulation developed, reaching its climax around 1979 and 1980. In the latter year, the Association of the British Pharmaceutical Industry was widely cited when it criticized the British Government for erecting 'a cumbersome and expensive regulatory edifice, much of which serves little useful purpose so far as the well-being of the public is concerned' (cited in[113]). During the four years since then, a series of major drug accidents (see Table V and Ref. 172) have caused opinion to swing again in favour of more extensive control. Not all these incidents would necessarily have been prevented by better drug control methods, but they have nevertheless been widely presented as reflecting the failure or limitations of current control mechanisms.

The source of the pressures influencing policies has not always been clear. Some universities and other apparently independent institutions involved in the debate have been commissioned by interested parties, primarily the pharmaceutical industry and bodies committed to promoting the interests of commercial enterprise, but sometimes also by political movements. Such sponsorship is commonly not made public, and it has not always been known even to policy makers. The material produced by such institutions is often accurate and useful, but it can at the same time be directed so unilaterally to matters of concern to the sponsor that it provides a misleading picture of the total situation.

One welcome recent trend is the greater degree of self-criticism among some of those involved in drug regulation, and by others working in industry, who have tried to identify and avoid certain of the adverse repercussions which their work might have. Griffin[34], though never sparing in his criticism of certain industrial practices, has pointed to the fact that the professional regulator may fall into various sins, including those of complacency, aloofness (or failure to communicate), rigidity of thought, pride and procrastination. All these can delay and complicate the regulatory process unnecessarily.

Table V[23, 123, 124, 146]   Suspensions and cancellations of licences for significant drugs in one or more European countries because of adverse effects.

(*March 1982 to February 1984*)

Benoxaprofen
Controlled release indometacin (Osmosin, Indosmos)
Oxyphenbutazone
Phenylbutazone
Zomepirac

Zimelidine
Althesin*
Propanidid*
Methrasone

---

*Because of content of Cremophor EL

2

Finding a methodical approach

1. THE GOAL AND THE MEANS

The whole point of studying regulation is that one hopes to find
ways of making it better. Naturally, we must not over-simplify;
in this field some perfectly genuine interests do conflict. One
should however at least try to define and measure these
interests so that they can be weighed openly against one
another at the political level.

Most of the facets of drug regulation listed in Table IV are
concerned with what Martin[76] calls 'social regulation', which is
concerned with 'standards for health and safety in the workplace, environment and products', and which is intended to
improve the quality of life. Another part of drug regulation in
the broad sense does however belong to the domain of
'economic regulation' (relating for example to patents, competition and monopolies). This book is concerned mostly with
the former area, and with work relating specifically to drugs. It
is important however to remember that the effects of both
social and economic regulation have been subject to a great
deal of study, particularly in the United States. Most of this
research has not been in the drug field, but one can learn from
it by analogy and adopt some of its methods[105].

Early studies of drug control usually provided mere comparisons of laws and regulations[66]. Others offered impressive
statistical overviews of regulatory activity which certainly
showed how busy the regulators had been but did not answer
the question as to whether they had been doing any good.

Hartley & Maynard[122] have correctly pointed to the fact that many types of data on regulation say nothing about its effects; they include accounts of the length and content of annual reports from regulatory bodies, the numbers of regulations and orders issued, the size of the regulatory staff, the number of inspection and enforcement activities carried out, the scope of post-marketing surveillance studies, the number of licences voluntarily withdrawn when products came up for official review and the number of changes made in testing procedures.

Comparative studies of the letter of the law and the regulations in different countries are again only of limited use. In a technical field such as this the legislator can lay down only the broad lines of an agency's activity; even new regulations and orders tend to trail behind actual practice. As one unanticipated problem after another arises the interpretation put upon the law and the regulations will be all-important. The harmonized legislation of the European Community, for example, can as pointed out earlier be interpreted in different ways in the member states, and if we are to study the effects of regulation we must study it as it functions in practice. A single example of interpretative differences may be taken from the cromolyn study in the European series. Although the written toxicological requirements of the various countries were similar, the assessors in two of the countries appeared to expect specific studies designed to exclude certain effects of cromolyn which might have been anticipated on theoretical grounds; those in other countries accepted the general toxicological work submitted by the manufacturer[71].

Over the last twenty years, the most substantial effort to analyse the effects of drug regulation, particularly on industry, has been made in the United States[105,133]. Much-quoted attempts to study the issue in the United States have been made by Peltzman[41], Baily[42], Jadlow[43] and Jondrow[44]. There have also been a long series of papers from the Center for the Study of Drug Development (Lasagna & Wardell)[45] as well as work by Grabowski[46] and by Schwartzman[47]. The controversy has been analysed further in seminars on pharmaceutical policy issues[38] and in overviews[90].

Despite the volume of this American material – and all the information which it provides – it has to be used with caution, if only because it relates to a situation which does not have an exact parallel anywhere in Europe. Much of the work has also been criticized on methodological grounds in the United States itself. Ashford has pointed out that 'the nature of the policy trade-offs has not been adequately defined, and the methodological approach to solving the trade-off problems has not been sufficiently developed. In the literature, anecdotes often substitute for data and value judgements are sometimes confused with analysis'[48]. In addition, the reservations expressed earlier in this chapter as to sponsorship by interested parties, such as the American Enterprise Institute, apply to a lot of the work. Exactly the same reservations have to be expressed as to some work published by some consumer groups on both sides of the Atlantic or by political parties[134], the starting point of which is sometimes opposition in principle to the activities of multinational companies. If in this review more criticism is to be found of material advanced by or sponsored by the pharmaceutical industry than by other parties, then this reflects only the fact that the greatest volume of work has emanated from that quarter.

Even the most elaborate approaches have sometimes fallen into methodological errors, as shown by various studies, reviewed by Ashford, of the effect of the 1962 amendments to American drug law. One such study by Peltzman[41] was founded on very basic and well-known concepts in the theory of demand, particularly the notion of consumer surplus. Ashford has argued that this concept is appropriate for the drug area only if several conceptual pitfalls are properly handled. Even then, he considers, its inherent limitations require a host of caveats and qualifications[48]. The same topic was later studied by two other groups. Baily[42], using regression analysis to study the effects of the 1962 amendments, and taking the post-amendment period as a dummy variable, obtained results indicating that the decline in new chemical entities per dollar spent on research and development was explained both by the depletion of research opportunities and by regulatory change. Grabowski *et al.*[72,82], applying multiple regression to additional observations and constructing a depletion variable based on pharmaceutical innovation in the United Kingdom, also showed a strong statistical relationship between the post-amendment period and a perceived decline in new chemical entities. Neither set of results support Peltzman's statistical conclusion that the amendments were *solely* responsible for the post-1962 decline in pharmaceutical innovation. Grabowski's study indeed suggests that a (cumulative) decline in new chemical entities per dollar spent on research and development existed for many years before 1962, thus again pointing to the likely influence of non-regulatory factors. A final criticism of the type of international comparison conducted by Grabowski could be that he did not find a common baseline; over a given period he detected a sixfold decline in the introduction of new chemical entities in the United States as compared with only a threefold decline in the United Kingdom, suggesting greater regulatory influence in the United States; however he advanced no evidence that the state of the pharmaceutical market and new drug introductions at the beginning of this period was comparable in the United States and the United Kingdom and there is reason to suspect that it was not.

Grabowski's work is only one of several early attempts to define problems with existing national systems by comparing them with others, but most such studies have been carried out to find support for a preconceived point of view, generally as regards the shortcomings of the U.S. Federal Food and Drug Administration. A 1980 report by the General Accounting Office, entitled: 'FDA drug approval – a lengthy process that delays the availability of important new drugs'[79] represents an official attempt to use the comparative method, but comments from members of the panel which reviewed the report raise serious questions as to the methods used[84].

Similar criticism can however also be levelled against many European papers on this issue, most of which, even if they purport to advance hard data, in fact represent special pleading on the basis of selected and anecdotal evidence. A typical paper by Burrell[35], suggestively entitled 'Drug assessment in uproar', provides such facts as the number of government forms filled out annually by Messrs Eli Lilly (apparently for all purposes combined) and the growth in the total number of government employees in the United States. Some papers have set out to ridicule drug control and drug controllers, just as others have sought to make the entire pharmaceutical industry appear unscrupulous.

Various fundamental fallacies are unfortunately to be found in a paper by Hartley & Maynard[122] which is often quoted for its view that in the United Kingdom a measure of deregulation or complete replacement of the existing structure by industrial self-regulation are desirable. In fact their conclusions emerge mainly from a wholesale rejection of arguments favouring regulation (which they regard as unproved), the prominence which they accord to the need for an economically strong industry, and their acceptance of hypotheses raised by others that the two are inconsistent. No distinction is made between artificial and generally accepted drug development standards, no attempt is made to check cause and effect relationships and no account is taken of transnational influences.

Fortunately, good work has been done sporadically on both sides of the Atlantic, and more of it has been done in the recent past. Preliminary work such as that produced so far by the Centre for Medicines Research in Britain[137] shows industry-sponsored studies at their best. Good independent work from the United States includes that of Ashford and his collaborators at the Massachusetts Institute of Technology, who have performed a series of balanced, though as yet incomplete, studies of the relationships between pharmaceutical regulation, innovation and therapeutic benefits[48, 49]. From 1980 onwards, the work of this group has been complemented by the World Health Organization's European Studies of Drug Regulation.

2. AIMS OF THE WHO EUROPEAN STUDIES OF DRUG REGULATION

Unlike much previous work, which concentrated mainly on the economic and scientific repercussions of drug control for the pharmaceutical industry, WHO's European Studies set out primarily to determine whether drug control as it currently functions in various parts of Europe is properly fitted to its basic purpose, i.e. the need to ensure that in drug matters the prescriber and the patient can be reasonably assured of efficacy, safety, quality and truth. Clearly, regulation must be considered to fail if the requirements set in any of these matters are either insufficient to protect the patient from harm or so exaggerated that the development or introduction of useful drugs is unnecessarily delayed or prevented.

This approach reflects the concept that, if these are the sort of guarantees which drug regulation is intended to provide, one should set out to find satisfactory ways of providing them (always allowing for human error and lack of knowledge). Having set the standards required, there should then be no compromises. If maintaining standards of efficacy or safety which have been shown to be necessary threatens investment or innovation in the pharmaceutical industry then other ways of protecting the latter must be found. These could involve direct research subsidies or tax relief; one could also envisage official efforts to promote transfer of technological information or extension of patent life so that innovation is adequately rewarded[80]. If the cost of the regulatory process threatens the development of drugs for rare diseases, then solutions for that problem too need to be found, such as the 'orphan drug' law now in operation in the United States.

This approach is to some extent theoretical since it is unlikely that one will be able to define and quantify all the facts or set ideal and agreed standards for every purpose; working in this way can however help to meet Ashford's objection to some earlier American work, namely that the 'policy trade-offs' have not been adequately defined.

Around this central approach a number of subsidiary approaches must be undertaken if we are to obtain a complete picture. One must examine all those secondary matters which are the subject of regulation in certain countries (e.g. prices, distribution – see Table IV) and all those repercussions of regulation which, whilst important, have a less direct effect on public health (notably effects on the industry itself).

The European Studies have so far concentrated on the effects of regulation in a number of countries which have relatively rigid systems, though it is clear that in attempting to define the optimum level of control one should look for situations of under-regulation and inappropriate regulation as well as over-regulation. The Studies have made much use of inter-country comparisons in order to provide control data for the situation in any given system, but without any preconceived idea as to which system may be 'preferable', if indeed one is better than another. Using the comparative method cautiously in an all-European context (with even broader comparisons where possible) can be rewarding, since the 32 countries of the WHO European Region differ so much in their regulatory traditions. They range from the relatively permissive approach found in parts of southwestern Europe to the much more restrictive traditions of Iceland and Norway and a surprising variety of approaches in Eastern European countries with a centralized economy.

In international comparative studies one inevitable question, already touched on in Chapter 1, is whether different populations do or do not need the same range of medicines. A reasonable hypothesis seems to be that although genetic, climatic, epidemiological and other variations need only lead to limited differences in the range of medicines needed between different populations there are at present much more strongly differing traditions in the use of medicines, largely for cultural reasons[57]. Cultural influences clearly can play a useful suggestive and placebo role in medical practice, and one could argue that a regulatory agency which tries to serve the community should allow for them; since for example the tradition of multiple prescribing is much stronger in Italy or France than in Denmark or Norway, the range of drugs and the number of fixed combinations may well need to be larger in the former countries than the latter, at least in the present state of society; for similar reasons, some marginally effective medicines traditional to a given country may have to be tolerated by the authorities there, but there is no reason to license them elsewhere. If this view is to be taken, there will be a fair range of variation in the 'optimal' situation from country to country, even within the limits imposed by the basic requirements of reasonable efficacy and safety; in international comparisons, therefore, one should be cautious about concluding that one policy is 'right' and another 'wrong'.

A very positive element in the European Studies has been their support by the WHO Regional Office for Europe. This independence of all interested parties, which brought with it a decision of principle to accept no funding from any of them, has provided the project team with a sound basis for action and proved of great value in opening doors which might otherwise have been closed. The main objection which might be advanced to the Studies is that they were initiated by drug regulators, who could be considered as seeking to defend their own professional activities. As in the case of other investigations however, the work must be assessed by the extent to which objectivity has been sought and is being attained.

3. FACTORS AFFECTING DRUG USE AND DEVELOPMENT

In trying to define cause-effect relationships in this area, problems unavoidably arise in studying regulation as an isolated causal element. It is too simple to conclude, as some writers do, that, because a change has come over the drugs field (or the health field more generally) since the introduction of a regulatory system, it must be a consequence of the latter. It is for example fallacious to present tables of declining mortality and morbidity in the present century as an integral part of the case for pharmaceutical innovation (see for example Wells[85]) unless one qualifies the link very carefully. To avoid fallacies like this, several important points will have to be borne in mind.

Firstly, many regulatory activities reflect the existence or emergence of a broad professional and consumer consensus on standards[54, 70]. In such cases, the lawgiver or regulator codifies the opinion of the community; he may also help to catalyse its development. Standards such as these would often be applied by ethically inclined pharmaceutical companies even in the absence of any regulation. As Ashford & Heaton put it: 'The perception by business of the need to change its technological course typically precedes the actual promulgation of a regulation'[105]. Naturally, the consensus itself may be wrong, but one must distinguish this question from that as to whether a regulatory agency has departed unreasonably from standards which are becoming generally accepted.

Secondly, the pattern of drug use and the drug market are probably largely determined not by drug regulation but by cultural traditions, initiatives taken by the pharmaceutical industry, the education and behaviour of prescribers, other governmental activities (such as patent legislation, taxation and economic policies, education and scientific research, which may develop concurrently with drug regulation) and by the whole structure of the health system.

Thirdly, drug innovation is similarly influenced by a series of interacting factors, which are reviewed elsewhere in this book. Ashford[48] finds for example broad agreement in the literature that the 1962 amendments to American drugs legislation were followed by some decline in innovative activity; however, both could have resulted, independently of one another, from such external influences as the thalidomide disaster in 1960-1961. The association could also have been coincidental, e.g. innovation could have reached a natural plateau at this time, such as has happened in some other fields; this view has also been cited by regulators in their defence of regulation[88]. May *et al.*[86], who found a marked reduction in the number of new chemical entities entering clinical testing, summarized a series of 'changes in both philosophy and the state of the art' which could have been responsible, alongside possible regulatory effects. It is also worth recalling that, well before the controversy around regulation developed, research directors in the pharmaceutical industry were quite aware of rapidly increasing research costs, which they attributed principally to 'new yardsticks of sophistication' which the 'new knowledge of . . . and increasing complexity of drugs' demanded[87].

The increased emphasis on both safety and efficacy has clearly changed the drug development process, for some firms quite dramatically, but one has to beware of using too coarse a measure. While the total number of new chemical entities may have decreased in the United States, for example, the significance of each therapeutic advance attained actually seems in some pharmacological areas to have increased[49]. Again, however, some of these changes might well have occurred independent of regulation[48, 105].

Grabowski *et al.*[94] in their comparison of productivity trends in the United States and the United Kingdom, held both the depletion of research opportunities and the increase in regulation responsible for the reduced productivity of drug research and development which they observed. Their regression analysis suggests for example that a (cumulative) decline in new chemical entities per dollar spent on research and development existed for many years prior to the Kefauver amendments to American drug law in 1962, thus pointing to the importance of non-regulatory factors in explaining part of the observed decline[48, 61]. Ashford *et al.* make the point however that in studies like this one should in fact break down all the data into suitably defined therapeutic areas, since both the causes and the effects seem to have differed from one field of medicine to another[48].

In a paper prepared for the National Science Foundation, Hansen[54] provides a useful discussion of the work of Jondrow, Baily and Grabowski as well as Peltzman. He concludes that no clear answer emerges from the work to date regarding the relationship between regulation or research depletion and the changes in pharmaceutical innovation.

Fourthly, just as regulation is only one of the factors affecting drugs, so drugs are only one of the factors which affect health statistics[136]. The general health level of the population, surgical techniques, nutrition and other elements are likely to have at least as great an effect on public health and to confuse the findings both nationally and in international comparisons.

Finally, the influence of national regulation has now become intermingled with that of foreign regulation. The actions taken by a regulatory agency of a large country can affect the research and investment policies of company based elsewhere; a multinational conglomerate company will indeed experience the combined effect of many different national policies, some of which are directly opposed to others. In addition, one regulatory body often influences the policies of another. The prolonged delay of the authorities in the United States and the United Kingdom in approving medroxyprogesterone acetate for use as an injectable hormonal contraceptive is well known; many importing countries were clearly influenced by these decisions[151], even though they were not generally followed on the European continent.

Communication between national regulatory agencies is, as pointed out in Chapter 1, now much more common than it was ten years ago. Positive decisions on new drug applications are now fairly rapidly announced internationally. Negative decisions are still, formally speaking, regarded as a matter which should remain confidential between the agency and the applicant; only Norway has taken the initiative to publish brief accounts of its drug refusals[142] though negative decisions taken elsewhere seem to be quite widely discussed between regulators on a personal basis. The pharmaceutical industry, apparently concerned as to the ripple effect of a negative decision taken nationally, has argued strongly that such measures should not be made known transnationally or that international communication should occur only after consultation with the manufacturer:

'First, every communication abroad by a national agency of regulatory or legislative actions should be approved at the highest possible level within the agency, and where practicable, by the head of the agency. Second, communications between agencies should consist of the facts only, with as much precision, background and detail as possible. As a corollary I would add that recipient agencies should not accept everything received at face value; they should request full details and bring their own judgements to bear.

Finally, the manufacturer should be consulted before communications involving its product are released. This is not only a matter of equity but also a means of enhancing accuracy, increasing information, and obtaining rapid co-operation, and it also provides the company an opportunity to discuss the confidential aspects of their material. This latter point hopefully would result in protection from the release of confidential information.'[116]

Transnational effects are naturally likely to be particularly strong in small landlocked countries with a limited regulatory apparatus of their own and considerable frontier traffic[119].

4. GETTING ACCESS TO THE DATA

Before one can even start to examine cause and effect in regulation, one must get hold of firm facts. The type of information which one needs will be discussed in Chapter 3, but right at the start one must make the point that getting objective data is not at all easy. One is trying after all to study dispassionately a field in which the debate has often been heated, with emotional overtones, and where there are many vested interests of an economic, political and personal nature. A major problem, already touched on, is the confidential nature of much of the relevant evidence. Even after regulatory agencies have learned to talk to one another they will be hesitant to provide any essential data to third parties. This is often understandable; a lot of regulatory activity relates to material which is unpatented and perhaps unpatentable, such as some aspects of research and of manufacturing 'know-how'. Drug regulatory agencies are for this reason bound by confidentiality clauses in law which prevent them from passing on to third parties information which they have received when dealing with applications. Even in those countries where freedom of information legislation has opened up official files to public scrutiny, special exceptions have been made for drug regulatory material.

Confidentiality clauses in fact often relate only to certain sensitive matters (e.g. pharmaceutical know-how) but they tend to be very broadly interpreted so that a manufacturer will not run the risk of seeing any type of information at all pass, via the regulatory agency, to a competitor[145]. This broad interpretation has been insisted upon by manufacturers[117] (see also above). For such reasons, most studies in this field have been dependent on very general information provided by one of the interested parties, which it has not been possible to supplement or verify. The European Studies have in this respect enjoyed a privileged position in that, as pointed out elsewhere, certain agencies and manufacturers have agreed to open their files to scrutiny; however, other agencies and companies have refused to do so.

5. APPROACHES TO THE PROBLEM

Determining the effects of a regulation is rather similar to determining the wanted and unwanted effects of a drug. Once we have excluded other causes, for example, reasonable proof that regulatory activity really has been responsible for a particular event will commonly depend largely on the time-sequence, except where a controlled (e.g. international comparative) study is feasible. As Cromie has written however[24], some of the ultimate effects of a regulation (like those of a drug) may take a very long time to be felt, perhaps 10–15 years. That certainly applies to effects on the pharmaceutical industry, but it can also apply directly in some areas of health care, e.g. where one is dealing with drugs used for long-term prophylaxis. This obviously raises the classic problem of any long-term study, namely that the baseline data may change during that period. Ashford, for example,[48] has pointed out that 'the level of drug development in the 1950s is often taken as the proper baseline representing the "no regulation" case, without adjusting for the complicating effects of other events or changes in the environment.'

Fortunately, there are instances where the effect of a regulation can be seen fairly rapidly. The history of the clinical trial certificate exemption scheme in the United Kingdom is a case in point. In the 1970s the pharmaceutical industry had repeatedly complained that the difficulty in obtaining clinical trial certificates in the United Kingdom was resulting in early clinical evaluation being conducted outside the United Kingdom, and studies by Griffin & Diggle[61] confirmed the fall in the number of certificates from 179 in 1973 to 87 in 1980. One aim of the exemption scheme which was subsequently introduced was therefore to stimulate early clinical evaluation of new drug substances. An increase in clinical trials was indeed achieved with 207 clinical trial expemtions being granted in the period 1 April 1981 – 31 March 1982, the number including studies with 76 new chemical entities. It is interesting however that by September 1982, 36 of these compounds had still not gone into clinical evaluation, i.e. 6 months or more after the granting of an exemption; in 14 of these cases the exemption had been granted more than 12 months before. Twelve of these products so delayed were new chemical entities. Five of the 36 products which had not commenced trial had been dropped for commercial reasons and two had faced problems with ethical committees which might have accounted for the delay. However for the remaining 29, including the 12 new chemical entities, no reason was given when the firm was specifically questioned[159]. It therefore appears that, despite efforts by the regulators to change the climate so as to facilitate clinical research, the industry was failing to maximise the opportunities offered to it[168]. As in other studies, one can see that where delays occur in matters subject to regulation they are not by any means always attributable to the fact that the regulations are there.

From much that we have said so far it is clear that the methods used in any impartial study of the effects of drug regulation have to be extremely well thought out; even the most honest work can easily be invalidated by confounding factors. Seven approaches which have been tried and tested are outlined below. Others which might be considered are described in Chapter 5.

(1) *International comparative studies of two or more regulatory systems which differ in some clear respect, looking at overall patterns but wherever possible also at appropriate sub-sets of data.* Studies of this type should provide data on the comparative efficiency of regulation, parallels and differences in decisions, and the effect of structural or legislative differences on these decisions.

An example of a preliminary study of this type is that by Lunde and Dukes[69] who in 1980 compared the overall regulatory tradition in the Netherlands with that in Norway. The Netherlands was a member of the European Community, Norway was not. Norway, unlike the Netherlands, has a 'need clause' in its legislation[12] which makes it possible to reject drugs regarded as unnecessary for medical practice. From each country a series of successive applications was examined which was large enough to include 100 consecutive negative decisions; this entailed studying 362 new drug applications in the Netherlands and 328 in Norway (taken over a comparable period of time). Aspects which were examined in this way

included the spectrum of applications coming in, the rate of
final rejection and reasons for rejection, the time taken to deal
with applications, and the differences emerging in all these
respects between innovative, semi-innovative and non-
innovative drugs. The results are discussed in Chapter 4.
Subsequent similar studies dealing with sub-sets of data are
those on non-steroidal anti-inflammatory drugs[50] and beta-
blockers[51].

Hass *et al.* have in a more superficial but broader study
provided a five-country comparison of the dates of introduction of new chemical entities on the market[78] which in part
reflects the speed of operation of regulatory systems.

(2) *Studies of the validity and effects of those specific measures
and policies which are contested by the pharmaceutical
industry and/or the medical profession, so that the entire
responsibility for their consequences can be considered to
lie with the regulatory agency.* The attractiveness of such
studies is that the causal effect can be isolated; one should
therefore be able to find out whether or to what extent a
law or a regulation has had unwanted effects, for example
on innovative capacity, industrial profitability and investment and whether it has produced any reasonable benefit
to public health.

Examples include certain long-term animal safety investigations studies and mutagenicity studies. Here one can calculate
the scientific capacity and funds occupied by this work and
make (at least in the long run) reasonable estimates of its
benefit or lack of benefit to society. The work of Walker *et
al.*[137] goes a long way towards reaching this ideal.

(3) *Studies of the purely national effects of a national regulatory system (or of specific measures within that system) on
industrial profitability, investment and innovation, in a
country where there is a substantial innovative industry
with a very large home market, so that transnational*

influences are very secondary. Although one will never exclude transnational influences completely, and the results are bound to be confounded by macroeconomic and other influences such work should again demonstrate the presence or absence of regulatory effects on innovative capacity, industrial profitability and investment.

Examples include existing studies from the United States and the United Kingdom; such work would also be feasible for some types of company operating in the Federal Republic of Germany and in Japan. Studies relating to the effects of a particular measure are for example those concerning the effect on industry of the 1962 Kefauver amendments to American food and drugs legislation.

(4) *Studies of the way a particular drug was handled by the regulators; these should preferably be carried out in collaboration with both the applicant and the agency, and if possible one should compare the course of events in one agency with that in others.* The evidence obtainable is the same as in approach (1) above, but it can be obtained in much greater detail so that the effects of particular acts on both sides can be impartially studied. One can, for example, study the ability of an agency to communicate clearly with the applicant and vice-versa. Such work can point directly to deficiencies in operation which, one may assume, will run counter to the direct public interest and the interests of industry.

An example is the cromolyn sodium study in the European series, which points to some of the advantages and drawbacks of different procedures within agencies[71]. 'This experience with cromolyn shows the value of a critical view of a file by individual experts, but also underlines the need for control on the work performed and the conclusions put forward by these experts. If a balanced and critically realistic view is to be formed, there is obviously great merit in according this work to committees, while not eliminating review by senior agency officials.'

One caveat in comparing the fate of a drug in the hands of different agencies is that one must also compare the files submitted; one agency may have received better documentation from the applicant than another.

(5) *Studies of the effect on incidence of specific types of drug-induced injury of restrictive measures taken on safety grounds in a specific country and not adopted elsewhere.* The evidence obtainable here is on the most efficient regulatory means of anticipating and preventing drug-induced injury.

A study in the European series of the validity of restrictive measures taken on safety grounds in Australia illustrates the possibilities of this approach[53]. It examined 50 consecutive major restrictive decisions (rejection, deferral or limitation) taken by the Australian agency, mostly on grounds of supposed safety problems (or inadequacy of safety evidence) over a total period of 27 months; the last of these decisions had been taken two years before the study was conducted. The problems considered to exist by the agency were then set against the subsequent literature to see whether they had indeed emerged in practice.

(6) *The study of effects on medical practice in a given country of specific regulatory measures generally conceived as reasonable and designed to influence prescribing.* Such work should provide evidence of favourable and unfavourable effects on prescribing and drug utilization; it should also detect instances where well-meant regulatory measures in fact have no effect at all.

Haaijer *et al.*[52] studied in this way the events which followed the registration of cimetidine in the Netherlands. It was approved only for certain indications for which the efficacy of the drug was considered to be proven. By questioning physicians, they examined the extent to which they nevertheless prescribed the drug for unapproved indications. In those countries where drug utilization data are available nationally it is of course relatively simple to detect the effects of certain types of regulatory measures, such as emphatic warnings to the profession, and Lunde & Lunde[143] have provided examples of these effects in the Norwegian situation.

(7) *Studies of the effects of regulation procedures on the quality of clinical trials in a country*. Such studies should provide evidence of any improvement in the scientific quality of drug research submitted to the regulatory authority over a period of years.

An example is a comparison which was made of the quality of studies submitted by companies for marketing authorization in France before and after modification of the regulations[153].

3

Data for studying drug regulation

1. PUBLIC DATA ON HEALTH

Having found some possible ways to study the effects of drug regulation, we must consider the various types of data on which they can be based. Much of this starting material is problematical; some is unreliable, some is inaccessible and a lot is only partly relevant.

Public health statistics are generally accessible and often internationally standardized (e.g. those relating to total mortality, morbidity, hospital admissions and costs of medical care). It is not however very likely that such broad parameters of public health will be affected to any detectable degree by drugs (and thus indirectly by drug regulation), at least in the short run. Drugs which dramatically change the outcome of disease, such as the most essential antibiotics, represent only a small proportion of the total and are likely to be available under any regulatory system. While the World Health Organization has estimated that some 200 drugs are enough to meet basic health needs, even the most restrictive of European countries – Iceland – has some 600 active substances on sale with 750 brand names and 1250 different forms. Most of the drugs to be found on any longer list represent mere alternatives, though some of them have secondary advantages. It follows that in a country with 2000 compounds in the form of 15,000 specialities that fact alone is not likely to result in any pronounced difference in public health statistics as compared with a country where only about 800 are on sale in the form of 2000 specialities (approximately the situation in Norway).

A better approach may be to take more specific public health parameters, preferably those which could be influenced by a particular drug or group of drugs. This will involve looking at a specific change in therapy and its direct medical and social consequences. For example, the replacement of barbiturates by benzodiazepines, which is largely a consequence of regulation, might be expected to have an effect on mortality from poisoning.

Work such as this probably needs a two-stage approach. In the first place, as Ashford has pointed out[48] one should consider 'those therapeutic and functional uses (and accompanying side effects) that would be achieved if a particular drug were correctly prescribed and appropriately administered, and not the benefits that are actually realized via the medical care delivery system.' The second stage involves getting data on real-world events relating to the drug. This would mean that, for example, phenacetin as such could in the first stage be considered an important, beneficial and safe drug; the reasons which led to its widespread prohibition many years after its introduction were a consequence of second-stage developments, i.e. prolonged over-use of phenacetin-containing analgesics, and not of any inherent shortcoming of the drug. Much the same holds good where a 'me-too' drug has come into widespread use as a result of heavy marketing without contributing anything new to health care. Second stage events such as public over-use or over-exuberant marketing are, if regulated at all, regulated in a different way to the first-stage event (i.e. licensing of the drug) and the role of regulation in the two stages needs to be looked at separately.

One type of information which is elusive but particularly intriguing is that on the public's state of health and well-being including the individual's own assessment of the quality of life and health he enjoys; many useful drugs probably have a clearer effect on such measures than upon the duration of a disease or the span of life. One can identify a large number of specific parameters relating to physical factors (disability, sleep, nutrition), social factors (family life, dependence) and emotions (distress, mental suffering) and methods have been developed to quantify some of them, but any such approach is bound to involve an extraordinary degree of effort.

'Health profiles' offer a less ambitious means of analysis. Their virtue, and weakness, is that they do not attempt to aggregate the various elements of information which they gather into a single score. Rather, as in the case of the Nottingham Health Profile, items such as mobility, pain experience, sleep quality and energy are simply presented as disparate variables for each subject. Shifts on any of these discrete scales may then be noted in relation to therapeutic inputs[27]. The practical value of such measures in assessing the importance of certain treatments (and thus of regulatory effects on these treatments) has yet to be tested. Ashford has developed other direct methods for evaluating the benefits of health and safety regulations. This work incorporates health quality models and other social science techniques which more fully capture the values of positive health outcomes[161].

Table VI Economic costs due to illness and injuries resulting from smoking, road traffic accidents and industrial accidents in Sweden 1970[28]
Units: Swedish Kronor (Millions)

Cause	Treatment costs	Production loss	Total
Smoking	90	410	500
Road traffic accidents	470	975	1,445
Industrial accidents*	161	850	1,011

*Including occupational diseases

A complementary approach involves measuring illness in

purely economic terms, and Jönsson[28] has outlined how it can
be done:

'The costs associated with disease or injury can be classified
into two principal categories: direct and indirect costs.
Direct costs represent the value of resources used to prevent,
detect, treat and rehabilitate the health impairment or its
effects. In practice direct costs are usually measured as
private and public expenditures for health services related to
a certain disease or injury. In addition there are often
non-health sector direct costs borne both by the patient and
others. Of specific importance are costs associated with
activities which have the purpose of avoiding the disease or
compensate for a certain impairment or handicap. However
important, these costs are usually not included in cost of
illness studies.

Indirect costs are the lost or forgone output of patients
suffering premature death or disability. This is normally
measured in terms of the wages that would have been earned
by these individuals if they had not had the illness. The
theoretical rationale for this is the human capital theory . . .
It is important (however) to be aware of the limitations of
the human capital approach. Health as an asset in itself, as a
consumption benefit, is not included in the estimation . . .
However, for description and explanatory purposes the
method can be accepted bearing in mind that the descrip-
tions and explanations will at best be partial'.

Published data involving the measurement of direct and indirect costs of ill-health and disease include a study of the
economic costs of motor vehicle injuries in Sweden and the
United States[29] and a comparison of the costs of illness due to
smoking, road traffic and industrial production[28]. The total
figures from the second of these studies are presented in Table
VI; the original analysis shows clearly that the indirect costs
predominate. Analogous approaches are being developed and
used to evaluate the economic effects of health care technology

in other fields[96] and these can equally well be applied to drugs.

The classic work with respect to the health economic effects of a specific drug has been done by (or for) the manufacturer of the first commercially available H-2 blocker, cimetidine, to examine the effects of such treatment on the costs and duration of treatment of peptic ulcer; the alternative (surgical) treatment is taken as a basis for comparison with loss of working time and hospitalization costs as important measures. Not surprisingly, this work has attracted a great deal of (sometimes critical) attention[96, 97, 101].

The general idea underlying the macroeconomic evaluation of cimetidine, as summarized by Jönsson[101], has been to start with a study of the economic costs of ulcer disease, continue with an *ex ante* study of the expected effects of cimetidine on these costs, and end with an *ex post* study of the actual effects of the introduction of the drug. Horisberger, in presenting some of the most optimistic conclusions to emerge from this work, calculated for cimetidine that 'the resultant net benefit for treatment of duodenal ulcer in the Federal Republic of Germany in 1980 amounts to DM 88.68 million'[98]. Bloom has however pointed to various shortcomings in such studies, mainly relating to the data base used[99]. Weisbrod has suggested that the difficulties in performing an entirely watertight cost/ benefit study will be insurmountable[97]; in his view, a 'useful' evaluation, which will inevitably be incomplete, should make clear the nature of its shortcomings and not hesitate to present non-monetary, quantitative measures of costs and benefits, leaving it to the user to decide upon their importance relative to other consequences.

Whether even an improved version of the cimetidine study will be suitable for wider use remains contentious. Sonnenberg *et al.*[100] have argued that cimetidine is a relatively simple case to evaluate because of the clear-cut distinction from the alternative forms of therapy. All the same, if one can find a reasonable compromise between perfection and simplicity and then extend this approach a little, it might be possible to examine the economic effects of a regulatory rejection of a 'breakthrough' drug or of a delay in its registration for a given period.

One should however bear in mind that economic measures of a drug's benefits only partially reflect the truth about it. Crout[110] has reflected what he finds to be the view 'of many health regulators that estimates of the health benefits and the health costs of a new drug, or a new regulation, are simply too subject to individual value judgements for such an analysis to have credibility.'

Finally, just as when dealing with social effects, one must be careful to look at both sides of the coin; if we are going to measure the social benefits produced by a drug we must also measure the amount of injury which it causes. Jönsson has also studied this latter question, adopting an economist's view of the costs of adverse drug reactions, calculated as the costs of other types of illness can be[28]. In order to adopt the approach already taken for the other forms of injury listed in Table VI, one would obviously have to limit the analysis to the more serious type of adverse reaction exceeding mere inconvenience and involving at least some loss of working time, and at most hospital admission, permanent disability or death. A problem here is clearly that we do not have the same knowledge of the epidemiology of adverse drug reactions as we have for road accidents, smoking and work injuries; quite apart from the fact that many reports of possible adverse reactions provide only a suspicion that a drug was responsible, many adverse reactions never get reported at all. Further, as Jönsson points out, most adverse reaction monitoring systems do not provide the data one needs for the calculations. As he puts it 'the description of the consequences of adverse drug reactions (ADR's) is very limited. It is possible to identify those cases where an ADR is the probable cause of death. It is also possible from the description of the nature of the ADR to get some information about the severity of the effect. But it is not possible to identify for example the medical expenditures or number of days lost from work due to ADR's.'

There is a little general information available, but it is

superficial and one figure contradicts the other. A Swedish study shows for example that 5.6% of hospital admissions were due to genuine adverse drug reactions[30]; a Swiss study shows a lower figure, namely 2%[31]. In purely practical terms, one has to agree with Jönsson that 'we today can't measure the direct and indirect costs of illness related to adverse drug reactions'[28] at least over a broad spectrum. It might be done for a few individual drugs, measuring the incidence and consequences of their adverse effects and then comparing these as between countries where regulatory policies have differed. Most agencies, when informed of drug problems arising elsewhere, will reflect on those which they have themselves succeeded in preventing or minimizing on their home ground by restrictive action, but as a rule such information will not be publicly available.

2. DATA ON REGULATORY AGENCIES

It is quite simple to define the sort of information about a drug control agency which one needs in order to study its achievements and its efficiency. One will need for example to know the numbers of applications and other matters dealt with and the outcome (with as detailed a breakdown as possible), the time taken to handle matters, and the grounds on which decisions were taken. In addition, figures on the actual cost of operating a regulatory agency obviously exist and should be open to scrutiny. As pointed out earlier, however, much of the scientific data internal to regulatory agencies is regarded as confidential and many agencies have too little staff to be able to free capacity for analyses of this sort.

A methodological problem is that agency terminology needs to be carefully standardized if comparisons are to be made and valid conclusions drawn. One agency may for example regard an application for the registration of a drug in both its oral and injectable forms as a single piece of business, others as two separate applications. Again, there are some countries, such as Belgium, where the raising of preliminary objections causes an application to lapse, and if the manufacturer later obtains new data he must submit a new application; in many other countries, such as the Netherlands, preliminary objections merely lead to suspension of the assessment until or unless a supplementary file is submitted. Such procedural differences need to be allowed for if they are not to distort international comparisons of acceptance and rejection rates.

The truth is sometimes hidden rather more deeply than one might imagine. Some companies, for example, will at an early phase of development of a drug submit a 'trial' application to test the reaction of agencies known to react quickly; such applications, which are very likely to be rejected, can again distort statistical analyses of regulatory activities. Again, the mere existence of a regulatory agency having a reputation for stringency may sometimes be sufficient to deter an applicant from submitting an application for a drug which is unlikely to meet its standards. This deterrent influence will only become apparent if one compares the numbers of applications actually submitted to various agencies, which differ markedly. Finally, the figures relating to certain agencies may be misleading unless set against the total background against which they operate. In the United Kingdom, for example, the total picture will emerge only if one considers data on applications dealt with by departmental staff, the more problematical applications sent for advice to the Committee on Safety of Medicines, and those going on appeal to the Medicines Commission.

Failure to standardize data collection in such respects explains the curious discrepancies in the literature between allegations that drug rejections are a rarity and analyses showing that negative decisions are quite common.

As with data obtained from the pharmaceutical industry, one must be watchful for bias in the selection and presentation of facts by official bodies; drug agencies have a position to defend.

3. EVIDENCE RELATING TO THE PHARMACEUTICAL INDUSTRY

It is important to distinguish between the research-based (generally multinational) pharmaceutical industry and firms occupied with generic manufacturing. Innovative companies can provide evidence on the capital investment and current expenditure required to meet the requirements set by regulatory agencies. In addition, the industry may be able, though more subjectively, to estimate to what extent the standards imposed by agencies differ from those which it would itself maintain in the absence of regulatory activity. Extrapolating from these data it may then be able to provide *estimates* of the effect of drug regulation upon its research programme, its total investments, and its turnover. A company can similarly report on the capacity and funds to repeat work from country to country in order to meet purely national requirements.

Evidence on concrete issues obtained from the pharmaceutical industry is generally well documented and quantified; a pharmaceutical company is likely to have more capacity available for extracting and presenting information of this type than will a regulatory agency. Limitations on the usefulness of these data are however imposed by the considerable differences between drug companies and the subjective nature of some of the evidence. It is for example not always easy for a company to provide a clear view on the standards which it would set for itself if only self-regulation existed. This may be feasible where, for example, quality control techniques are concerned, but it will be much more difficult with respect to most data on safety; standards on this latter matter are determined only in part by scientific conviction; they are attributable in part to the desire to demonstrate that all reasonable steps have been taken to ensure safety despite doubt as to the validity of the methods available; what is more, the standards advocated by a drug company are likely to have been influenced considerably by its past dealings with agencies, even if it is not fully conscious of the fact.

In interpreting evidence on the pharmaceutical industry's overall situation one must also beware, as pointed out in an earlier section, of attributing all its problems to the advent of drug regulation. Particularly the expiry of many important patents during the last two decades, the increase in the cost and complexity of innovative research, the long economic recession and the growing importance of generic manufacturing companies (sometimes operating in low-cost areas of the world) are undoubtedly responsible in large measure for problems which innovative industry experiences.

Finally, with Ashford's group[49] one must be cautious in handling any sort of evidence bearing on a wide and heterogeneous range of products; particularly where studies of innovation are concerned one must examine the effects of regulatory and other influences on specific sub-categories of drugs. As they point out 'Therapeutic areas are (1) differentially affected by the various regulatory actions, (2) subject to a different trade-off between efficacy and safety, (3) in a different stage of technology evolution, (4) administered differently by physicians, (5) dependent to a varying extent on government research, and (6) subjected to a different amount of market competition.'

Evidence on innovative activity   In any field, invention has to be distinguished from innovation[105]. In the process of drug development, the mere creation of a new compound is often not truly innovative from the medical point of view, but even where it is not it may be followed by a chain of innovative events. Any assessment of external effects on successful innovative activity (as opposed to the mere volume of the research effort) will therefore involve studying the process towards its end-point and choosing an appropriate unit of measurement.

The most readily available, though far from ideal, measure of innovative activity is the number of new chemical entities being developed or (preferably) reaching the stage of clinical testing or marketing. Reis-Arndt, for example, noted a fall in the number of new chemical entities introduced annually at some place in the world from 93 in 1961 to 48 in 1980 (quoted by Wells[85]). Similar figures (with a fall from 89 to 35 annually over a 21-year period) have been noted by Wardell's group for the numbers of new chemical entities entering clinical testing in the United States[86]. In the United Kingdom, Ravenscroft & Walker[164] noted a decline in the rate of introduction of new chemical entities from about 50 or 60 in the early 1960s to about 25 per annum between 1964 and 1967 with about 20 marketed each year for 1968 to 1982.

Even with this simple measure errors can arise unless we decide in advance what constitutes a new chemical, e.g. whether a new ester or salt of an existing compound should be so classified. It is however also clear that merely to count new drugs entering the market or the clinic is not a sufficient measure of successful innovative activity, since the quality as well as the quantity of innovation matters. Lunde & Dukes[69] developed for the European Studies a rating of innovation which has since been applied in various investigations by themselves and others (Table VII). It can be used either to classify the degree of innovation which the manufacturer claims at the time of submission (which may flatter the outcome but helps to eliminate investigator bias) or the investigator's own view of the innovative element in a given drug.

An alternative scale, with a five point rating for chemical originality and another five point scale for rating the degree of innovation, has been developed by the U.S. Federal Food and Drug Administration for its own studies. The scale proved to be insufficiently detailed for the European Studies and included some elements (e.g. status under 'DESI' or 'OTC' review) which were applicable only to one regulatory system. Whatever the classification used, it should enable one to study the qualitative as well as the quantitative effects of regulation upon new drug introductions, as well as differentiating the fate of applications for drugs at different levels of innovation.

Clearly there are other ways of measuring innovative activ-

ity; one can classify the novelty of the molecular structure or
the pharmacological action or study the number of patents
issued, the number of screening tests performed, the market
performance of new drugs, or the numbers of publications
relating to them. All these and others have been proposed by
Wardell[73] but most of them can be quite irrelevant to the public
interest; they may for example be useful to industrial management in determining the commercial productivity of an individual research unit in terms of the sales resulting from a given
volume of scientific effort, but even then they should probably
be used to complement rather than replace measures of clinical
innovation since this is the most solid basis for commercial
success as well as for public benefit.

Nor are changes in the number of companies engaged in
innovative research all that informative; Grabowski[91] attaches
some importance to the 'seemingly paradoxical' finding that
the number of such companies in the United States has fallen,
but in a multidisciplinary field such as pharmaceuticals an
increasing concentration of research into fewer but larger units
is only to be expected, irrespective of regulatory influence.
Similar considerations apply to the fall in the number of firms
introducing new products[103].

Agreement on the extent of innovation in the drug industry
and the sources of innovation is in fact lacking, though it is
widely considered that only a very small proportion of the new
and modified drugs entering the market in fact represent
medically important advances[70]. The FDA scale provides a
more generous estimate of true innovation than most clinical
pharmacologists would accept; on this basis some 50–60% of
new chemical entities were considered to constitute a therapeutic gain, ranging from 'modest' to 'very important'[111]. In a
comparison of applications in Norway and the Netherlands,
Lunde & Dukes[69] found that even if one accepted the applicant's view of the degree of innovation which his product
represented, only some 10% of applications in either country
could be regarded as innovative; approximately half the applications in either country were not claimed by the companies

in question to have any innovative element at all.

Table VII Classification of new drug applications according to innovational element (Modified from Lunde & Dukes, 1980[69]).

---

1. *Fully innovative submissions*

   A   New chemical compounds claimed to have novel fields of application, novel mechanisms of action or other substantial advantages over current products.

   B   Preparations designed for novel fields of application, documented by original research though the compound used is not new.

   C   Novel types of combinations, claiming to serve new purposes and documented by original research.

   D   Pharmaceutical innovations claimed to be of substantial practical importance in therapy.

   E   Other innovations claimed to be of substantial novelty and importance.

2. *Semi-innovative submissions*

   A   New chemical compounds belonging to existing therapeutic groups (irrespective of whether they are structurally novel or not) without clearly novel elements in their claims ('Me-too').

   B   Pharmaceutical innovations claiming to represent minor advantages (e.g. duration of action, convenience of use, or lower cost).

   C   Fixed combinations ⎫
   D   Herbal remedies   ⎬ claiming to represent minor advances.
   E   Infusion fluids   ⎭

   F   Other semi-innovative submissions.

3. *Non-innovative submissions*

   A   New brands of existing compounds.

   B   New forms of dosage strengths of known* compounds**.

   C   Fixed combinations ⎫
   D   Herbal remedies   ⎬ of an entirely traditional type.
   E   Infusion fluids   ⎭

   F   Other non-innovative submissions.

---

* i.e. already on the market in the country concerned.
** If advantages are claimed in terms of safety or efficacy (rather than mere convenience) code as 2B.

The pharmaceutical industry can naturally also provide detailed accounts of its experiences with regulatory agencies. In particular it can give evidence on their behaviour – their openness and helpfulness (or lack of it) – and assess whether their officials are realistic in their demands and in touch with current scientific trends. Industry can perform useful analyses of the relevance and irrelevance to man of particular types of experiment (e.g. long-term animal studies) on the basis of extensive and often unpublished data. Again, guidelines issued by different authorities yet all applicable to the same problem can be compared and any significant differences identified.

Until recently industrial companies have generally been reluctant to provide detailed information on their regulatory experiences, especially where named agencies and products were involved, for fear of either divulging industrial secrets or deranging the relationship with the agencies concerned. There is clearly in any case a need for verification of the statements made. There are also practical problems such as the fact that a company's regulatory experiences with a single product may be scattered over many offices in different countries, so that a great deal of work will be involved in collecting the relevant records, possibly translating them, and then collating and assessing them. Furthermore it is important that the view of the agencies on the points which arise should be obtained and discussed. The collaborative studies discussed below provide a partial solution to these problems.

4. EVIDENCE FROM PHYSICIANS AND THE PUBLIC

The practising *physician* is often not conscious of regulatory influences on his work, but he can provide evidence which will be useful in determining the effects of drug regulation on his prescribing. On the one hand, he can often supply figures on his therapeutic practices (drug utilization data); on the other he is a useful source of opinions if specifically questioned.

Dukes & Lunde, in one of the European Studies, obtained data on the prescribing of antirheumatic drugs by physicians in

Norway, as well as a statement of their preferences and their views as to whether the range of drugs permitted on the national market was adequate to meet their needs[50]. A subsequent study in the series provided evidence on physicians' use of (and preferences for) beta-blockers[51]; Haaijer and others were able to analyse the extent to which physicians in their prescribing followed the list of indications approved by a national regulatory agency[52].

Specific studies of the type needed to elicit physician-based data are labour intensive but valuable in checking directly the influence of a regulatory agency and the extent to which it is meeting the needs of the medical community. The (controversial) view cited in Chapter 1 that delay in the approval of beta-blockers for important indications in the United States led to deaths on a large scale could easily have been checked by asking practitioners which alternative treatments they were using at that time and how effective they were.

Although the practitioner is in most respects an intermediary between the regulatory agency and the public, there is a direct confrontation in certain fields. The *public* can provide evidence on matters such as the adequacy and comprehensibility of directions folders and packaging texts approved by regulatory agencies; it can also express views on the adequacy of the list of drugs permitted for self-medication. Some of this evidence may be obtained from organizations claiming to represent the consumer though these vary very much in their competence and standards. Some are composed of patients with a specific disorder and these organizations are often well informed and able to offer constructive comments. Others are groups of victims and alleged victims of some drug 'catastrophe', and may exert much pressure on regulatory agencies. Still others represent anti-doctor or anti-industry pressure groups. One must thus select one's organization carefully. For some purposes, it will be better to approach the public directly. Haxthausen, in a preliminary study for the World Health Organization, has in this way obtained facts and views on drug information, using street interviews[63].

5. OTHER SOURCES OF DATA

The collaborative approach   A problem already mentioned several times is that of confidentiality. An approach which has proved successful as part of the European Studies of Drug Regulation has been the study of regulatory files by an impartial third party (the WHO project team); some regulatory agencies and certain companies proved willing to open their records for study of a specific issue, the condition being that the other party would do likewise. The WHO team's methods have for the first time rendered it possible to examine the course of events in some major applications for new drug registration, using data from both sides to obtain a balanced view. Collaborative studies are likely to be the only valid means of studying the vexed question of regulatory delay which is often attributable to faults on both sides. So-called delay can indeed be due to the inefficiency or overloading of an agency but it can also result from inadequacy of the application or the slowness of an applicant in replying to reasonable questions.

The need for this approach clearly emerges from the short-comings of even well-documented evidence from a single party. One much quoted case relates to the drug Hyperstat (diazoxide), developed in the United States by the Schering Corporation. Patented in 1961, its New Drug Application was submitted to the United States authorities in 1963, and not given final approval until ten years later, i.e. five years before the patent was due to expire in 1978[47]. This appears to have been a classic example of new regulations unreasonably en-snaring an obviously useful drug which had been developed before the general introduction of requirements on controlled clinical trials[160], but one wishes that this case could have been studied with all the files open; it would certainly have proved instructive.

The collaborative method used in the first completed collaborative study of this type, that relating to cromolyn sodium, may be taken as an example. Here, the project team of the European Studies concluded separate agreements with the manufacturer of cromolyn on the one hand and with five regulatory authorities (those of the United States, Canada, Norway, The Netherlands and Sweden) on the other. A sixth (European) agency was in fact approached but did not feel able to supply information in view of its policy of maintaining complete confidentiality, even though no objection was raised by the manufacturer. All parties provided the team with a detailed history of the registration of cromolyn sodium in its original form in these countries. The histories were supplemented by copies of essential documents in the company's possession, including correspondence with the regulatory agencies. After analysis of the material, certain supplementary information and relevant comments were requested from all parties. In three countries it proved desirable to examine the agency's file directly. The analysis made was submitted to all the participants and in the light of the comments received a final text was compiled. The comments did not result in the deletion of any facts or of any criticism; they did however very clearly lead to a better insight into various matters and the correction of some errors[71]. The final analysis provides a striking picture of the best and the worst in drug regulatory practice.

The *medical and epidemiological literature* is likely to be the ultimate arbiter of the value and safety of a drug, matters on which it may not be possible to take a definitive view until · many years have passed. Since the effects of drug control are exerted (and have to be studied) over a very long period, a very long-term view can and must be taken. If a new drug or class of drugs substantially affects mortality, morbidity, the duration of illness, the length of hospital stay, or if it produces long-term injury, this should ultimately be evident from the literature unless it is obscured by interfering factors. As is evident from examples cited earlier, however, literature data on these matters can be grossly misused and it is rarely so complete in the short-term view that one can draw conclusions from it. The literature is also likely to prove most useful in identifying a medical consensus on a particular issue, against which the acts and standards of regulatory agencies can be tested[53, 68].

Evidence on *drug quality standards* can be relevant to the study of regulation. The quality of drug formulations influences their absorption, effects, adverse reactions and elimination; excipients, degradation products and packaging materials may all affect efficacy or safety. Although research-based manufacturers and many reputable companies manufacturing generic products undoubtedly do maintain high and consistent quality, it is clear when one examines samples submitted during tendering that there are secondary manufacturers whose standards leave a lot to be desired. Two factors that must also be taken into consideration are the extent to which drug production complies with the accepted rules of good manufacturing practice as outlined in WHO recommendations and how far the quality is in accordance with accepted norms such as those set in the pharmaceutical inspection convention or the standards and protocols of the European Community (EEC Directive 75/318).

We do not know at present how extensive these quality problems are, where they are to be found or how successful drug regulatory agencies have been in containing them. Evidence on pharmaceutical matters such as this could point the way to a proper balance of regulatory priorities. In a country where a larger number of products from secondary manufacturers are on sale there may be much greater justification for an extensive quality control apparatus within the regulatory authority than in other countries where the greater need is for evaluation of efficacy and safety or of promotional material.

Finally, *drug utilization data* can be of very great importance in determining to what extent regulation influences the prescribing and use of pharmaceuticals. Surprisingly enough, such data are in many countries not readily available and industrial surveys providing such figures are regarded as confidential. Fortunately, the work of the WHO Drug Utilization Research Group has in the last decade done a great deal to improve this situation. Utilization data must however be set against reliable figures on the numbers of drugs available in order to obtain a complete picture; Finland has for example a larger number of fixed analgesic combinations on its market than does Norway, but the utilization of such products is nevertheless higher in the latter country[155].

4

Current studies and findings

1. THE PRINCIPAL EFFECTS

Indicators of health and illness As pointed out earlier, there are only limited possibilities for identifying a correlation between drug regulatory policies and broad parameters of public health, but some links may be identified. The classic series of studies measuring correlations between a drug and a public health issue were those on cimetidine already described in Chapter 3, though they were conducted largely in economic terms. From the strictly regulatory point of view one could, if one were to accept the conclusions of these studies, calculate the public health effects of a delay in the registration of this preparation. In actual fact there does not appear to have been a marked regulatory delay in the registration of cimetidine even in countries with relatively restrictive policies. Hass *et al.*[78] cite as marketing dates in the United Kingdom 1976, in France, the United States and the Federal Republic of Germany 1977 and in Italy 1978. Data available to the Project Team indicate the date of registration in Norway as August 1978. The main differences in registration dates appear to have been due to differences in the dates of submission, and some difference of opinion as to whether the drug could be released so long as human efficacy and safety data were available only for short-term treatment.

It would be more instructive to analyse those cases where a serious regulatory delay is stated to have occurred in one or more countries for a drug of similarly innovative character. Again, although the remarkable allegation cited earlier that delay in the acceptance of certain claims for propranolol cost the lives of a quarter of a million Americans does not deserve serious consideration, any verifiable allegation of this type for a life-saving drug could provide a means of measuring the consequences of unjustifiable regulatory delay.

Drug standards The most basic question of all is whether drug regulation achieves its declared purpose, i.e. of protecting the public against ineffective, unsafe, or inadequately studied drugs. An absolute answer would require a more complete view of rejected new drug applications than is ever likely to be obtainable, but comparative studies, particularly in the European series, give some clear pointers. One cannot merely assess the degree to which a regulatory agency is serving the purposes set for it by counting the drugs on the market, as some have sought to do, since medical views on the range of drugs required to meet health needs can, as pointed out earlier, differ from country to country. By digging a little deeper, one can however obtain some evidence.

A first approach relates to *acceptance and rejection rates*, which should throw light on the view sometimes advanced that registration is a mere bureaucratic formality. In their first comparative study, between Norway and the Netherlands, Dukes & Lunde found rejection rates averaging at least 28% in the Netherlands and 30% in Norway[69]. The reasons were largely lack of clinical proof of efficacy and safety, though the conclusions as regards the clinical data were often supported by the evaluation of the findings in animal studies. Attempting to determine whether the fault lay with the drug itself or with the documentation presented, these investigators presented the subjective conclusion that in at least 27 of 100 rejections the file on a basically acceptable drug had been poorly prepared (i.e. the investigations were probably inadequate) and that in at least 58 of these 100 cases the drug itself would not have attained the requisite standard, even if it had been further investigated.

Very similar rejection rates have been noted from the United Kingdom by Griffin & Diggle[61], though their approach was not exactly identical. During the period 1979–1980, a total of 488 product licence applications were referred to the Committee on Safety of Medicines. The proportion receiving 'notice of S21(1) action' (pending rejection) rose from 28.2% in 1978 to 65.0% in 1980. These data do however need some further explanation. The 'licensing authority' is in fact the body primarily dealing with applications; it only refers to the Committee for advice those applications which relate to new chemical entities or novel products, or those which it is 'minded to reject'; the Committee figures on rejection rates are thus not strictly comparable to those from other countries which relate to all applications received. By 1984 the rejection rate at Committee level had at all events risen further to approximately 80%[168].

Data collected by Lunde & Bayer for Hungary show a 23% rejection rate over an 11-year period[65]. In Iceland, which bases its drug decisions partly on evaluation protocols from some other Nordic countries, Kristinsdottir found a rejection rate ranging from about 12% to 30% per year during the period 1977 to 1981[118].

Similar figures can be found when studying individual therapeutic groups. In a subsequent European study[50], the number of non-steroidal anti-inflammatory drugs marketed in a range of European countries in 1980 was found to range from 7 in Norway and 11 in Czechoslovakia to 50 in Italy. A number of other countries occupied a median position with 20–30 products on sale, the spectrum in these countries being very similar. Since the range of drugs marketed only in Italy comprises largely the products of internationally based companies, it would seem reasonable to conclude that many had been rejected elsewhere. Data available to these investigators on their work in the Netherlands and Norway confirmed this conclusion; 10 of 15 applications for such substances had been rejected in Norway and 9 of 18 in the Netherlands.

While figures such as these do not prove that the relatively restrictive policies in Northern Europe are correct policies, the fact that closely similar decisions were taken by national agencies working largely independently of each other indicates a broad consensus that for one reason or another the drugs rejected did not merit approval. Such data and others cited with respect to restrictive decisions certainly discredit the view that registration is today a mere formality; the estimate made by Dench, writing for the pharmaceutical industry (as quoted by Wells[85]), that once a product has reached a regulatory agency the chance of its being marketed has risen to 95% is apparently not in accordance with the facts, unless we limit the analysis to the very small number of drugs which can be regarded as fully innovative[61].

Another basic question relates to the *extent to which old drugs, on sale before an agency was established, have subsequently been assessed by it.* In the Netherlands, one of the first countries to undertake such retrospective assessment, more than 2000 of 5000 'old' drugs had been assessed within 10 years of the establishment of the agency in 1963, probably a record for any country. Unhappily, after the Benelux agreement in 1973 formally transferred responsibility for this work to an intercountry agency[130] the latter failed to continue it (simply because of the workload); the number of outdated and un-evaluated drugs on sale in the Netherlands has recently been the subject of criticism[70].

Some workers, concerned with what they regard as over-lenient regulation, have examined the *proportion of drugs marketed which subsequently have to be withdrawn for reasons connected with efficacy and safety.* Steward & Wibberley[113] used this method in the United Kingdom. Over 20% of the new chemical entities introduced before the Committee on the Safety of Drugs started operation, were subsequently with-drawn from the market. After 1964 there was a very much lower rate of withdrawal, falling to about 2% by 1972–1975. However, their findings do show some oscillation in the withdrawal rate over successive three-year periods, and in view of shifts in regulatory policy such a study needs to be continued over a long period to provide valid results. One could for example try to determine whether the new wave of drug withdrawals which was noted during the period 1982–1984[70, 172] was in any sense a consequence of relaxation under pressure of regulatory standards during the preceding years.

Effects on prescribing If regulation markedly affects the range of drugs it will also in this way affect prescribing; beyond a given point, it could impair the physician's ability to treat his patients adequately. One can and must therefore study directly the extent to which the current range of drugs in a particular country meets prescribers' perceived needs. This point has been investigated as regards non-steroidal agents, comparing the situation in the Netherlands where, by 1980, 22 products had been admitted to the market, with that in Norway where only 7 such products were available[50]. All practising rheumatologists in the two countries were approached.

In the Netherlands 45 rheumatologists provided data. The average rheumatologist was found to be using some 12 or 13 of the 22 products on sale, but the number he used regularly was much smaller, the mean being 6.60 ($\pm$2.33, SD). This did not mean, however, that six or seven drugs fulfilled most needs, since the actual choice of 'favourite' drugs varied quite markedly between rheumatologists, and even minor products had their protagonists. The figures suggested that if any attempt were made to limit the number of compounds to less than about 15, much professional opposition would be encountered. Although the attention of rheumatologists was drawn to the fact that more than twice as many non-steroidal anti-inflammatory agents were available in Italy as in the Netherlands, none of the doctors remarked that their choice was too limited. The Central Inspectorate for Medicines, which can make foreign drugs available to practitioners on special licence if requested, had in the course of two years received (and granted) only one such request for a non-steroidal anti-inflammatory drug not available in the Netherlands. In Norway, corresponding data were obtained from 44 rheumatologists. The average respondent was using 4–6 of the 7 drugs available, the pyrazolone derivatives largely being avoided. Of the rheumatologists responding, 25% commented that a wider range of drugs should be available in this field. No less than 40% of rheumatologists were found to be making occasional use of foreign drugs imported on special licence, and 363 such licences for these drugs were granted in the course of a year.

The investigators recorded their impression that some 10–15 of the currently existing non-steroidal anti-inflammatory drugs should be available to meet the need of rheumatologists. This would mean that the range of drugs allowed on the market was more than generous in the Netherlands but too restricted in Norway. This impression seems to be reflected in another study from the Netherlands, performed by Wierenga and relating to beta-blockers; 75% of Dutch general practitioners and internists providing comments considered that the number of beta-blockers on the market was excessive, and 50% of cardiologists were of the same opinion[51].

Data collected by Hemminki[120] also seem to show that the number of special licences issued is roughly proportional to the stringency of the regulatory system. Comparing four Nordic countries she noted that, in 1977, 1,971 special licences were issued in Denmark, 1,424 in Finland, 16,189 in Norway and 27,802 in Sweden. Since the Swedish figure includes more than 10,000 licences for special foods, the parallel is quite striking.

It has become clear however that one can interpret the data on special licences in various ways. In the European Studies cited above the view was adopted that the special licensing procedure appeared to be a reasonable measure to meet the needs of the individual patient where these were not satisfied by the entire procedure, which she regards as over-used and capable of defeating the purpose of drug regulation by in effect pampering to the whims of the individual physician. The views expressed in this paper have been criticized, not least because the number of special licences issued in Sweden or Norway is still only a negligible fraction of all prescriptions written. Nor can it generally be regarded as an aim of regulation to set aside entirely the judgement of the individual practitioner. The procedure in use in the Netherlands to assess requests for special licences, requiring the physician to provide at least some documented argument for considering that the drug which he wishes to import will indeed meet a particular need, might provide a simple means of avoiding abuse of the procedure. The question of special licensing is however certainly one which will merit impartial study if the volume of trade through this channel ever becomes excessive.

In future studies of regulatory effects on prescribing, one might need to be a little more cautious about using the opinions of practitioners as a means of defining objective needs. Certain widespread prescribing habits and expectations with respect to drugs seem to have grown up without any good reason (e.g. the belief that the ageing heart needs digitalis as a tonic) and some may be fostered by deliberate want creation. Even the view, cited in one of the above studies, that a fair range of drugs is needed for the management of rheumatoid arthritis, can be and is challenged. In that paper the authors stressed that even in 1980 there were authorities who considered that none of the current non-steroidal anti-inflammatory drugs could really equal aspirin, and the same view pertains in some quarters in 1984[144].

Quite another question is whether regulators have a more direct effect on prescribing practice. Some agencies are authorized by law to communicate directly with physicians (e.g. by issuing bulletins or newsletters); the influence of such activities does not seem to have been studied. All agencies are however involved in checking, amending and approving data sheets, directions folders or analogous documents for approved drugs, relating to such matters as indications, dosage, contraindications, adverse reactions and warnings. These texts are generally available to physicians in collected form as compendia, issued free of charge.

Present evidence does not suggest that the influence of the agencies in this respect is at all comparable with that of the pharmaceutical industry's travelling representatives. A paper in the European series by Haayer *et al.*[52] showed that of the prescriptions issued by general practitioners in the Netherlands for cimetidine, more than half were apparently being issued for indications not approved by the Netherlands Drug Regulatory Agency. Although, if one considered the entire range of possible indications for the drug, practitioners tended to use it for those approved by the Agency, the fact that some of the non-approved indications related to very common medical conditions explained the high proportion of prescriptions for such purposes. Again, in the United Kingdom an epidemic of deaths in intensive care units was traced to the use of the drug etomidate in a manner not authorized by the Committee on Safety of Medicines[168]. Another Dutch paper by Wieringa found similarly that beta-blockers were widely used for indications which had been rejected by the control agency, notably the treatment of nervousness[51].

By contrast, and as pointed out earlier, Lunde & Lunde have identified clear effects on Norwegian prescribing of emphatic warnings and other measures emanating from the regulatory agency[143], and it is not impossible that acute measures of this type have much more influence on the physician than the general body of regulatory decisions. Similarly, the 'Dear doctor' letters sent to all physicians by drug regulatory agencies in the United States, the United Kingdom and other countries, appear to have been successful in drawing prescribers' attention to new adverse effects, important changes in the range of indications approved for a drug, partial or total recall of a product and suchlike[168, 173].

This entire question of the effect on doctors of data sheets and other material carrying agency approval certainly needs much more careful study. Whilst the views of an agency are not always beyond dispute, they are based on more documentation than the practising physician is ever likely to see. The matter is of great practical importance. Several instances are known of drugs which were accepted for an indication of negligible importance, only to be prescribed subsequently on a vast scale for other (and unproven) indications. If this happens very often, it defeats much of the purpose of the regulatory system.

Effects on drug-induced disease Although, as pointed out in Chapter 2, methods can be developed for measuring the effects of regulation on drug-induced injury, very little work has so far been done to this end. One preliminary study is that in the European series relating to the Australian situation. This study, carried out in Australia because of that country's excellent system for recording regulatory decisions in detail, examined 60 adverse reaction problems which had been identified by the agency and which underlay 50 restrictive decisions. In the light of subsequent literature, 32 of these problems proved to have been correctly anticipated; in 6 cases the agency's prediction of a problem was marginally correct and in 5 cases it was wrong. In 17 cases no conclusion was possible, largely because long-term problems were concerned[53]. These restrictive decisions had been taken over a period of only 27 months, and one must add to them a much larger number of restrictions imposed upon data sheets and packaging inserts, most of which may have helped to prevent drug-induced injury. This type of study can thus profile the extent to which a national agency has indeed succeeded in reducing drug-induced disease and the cost and effort involved in doing so.

Alongside regulatory actions which anticipate and prevent adverse effects one can also examine the extent to which authorities have been successful in detecting adverse reactions with existing drugs and taking steps to limit or arrest iatrogenic epidemics. The detection of adverse effects falls outside the scope of this book, but it is not difficult to study major restrictive decisions on existing drugs, including the suspension and withdrawal of licences, because of adverse effects. During the biennium preceding the writing of this book, a succession of major products from international research-based companies were withdrawn from the market in some or all countries as a result of such regulatory measures (Table V). Depending on one's point of view, corrective measures such as

these can either be regarded as evidence of the need for
regulatory activity (and the failure of self-regulation) or as
reflecting the failure of current regulatory techniques to detect
and prevent problems such as these at an early stage. As
Offerhaus has put it, in a discussion of several such events:

> 'One must ask oneself how it is possible that such drugs ever
> succeeded in reaching the market. All the countries in which
> these drug catastrophes occurred have respectable and re-
> spected drug regulatory agencies, yet these apparently did
> not function properly. Could such events not have been
> prevented? The answer must be: in part. On the one hand
> there was apparently insufficient awareness that this sort of
> disaster could still occur, on the other hand the relative
> incidence of life-threatening or fatal reactions proved to be
> so low that they could never have been discovered in the
> clinical studies prior to registration, which as a rule encom-
> pass only a few thousand patients.' (Quoted in translation)[70]

Jönsson[28] has suggested that one should set the costs of adverse
drug reactions (ADR) against the costs incurred in preventing
such drug reactions, to determine whether there is a reasonable
balance. From a theoretical point of view, as he argues, one
should seek to find the point where the sum of the costs of
adverse reactions and the costs incurred in avoiding them has
its minimum. This concept, outlined in Figure 1, could be
useful in attempting to determine whether existing policies
have resulted in a situation to the left or to the right on the
curve, i.e. where the costs of prevention have become dispro-
ortionate to the size of the problem or the expenditure on
prevention is grossly inadequate to help in reducing the costs
resulting from adverse effects. The approach is logical, provided one continues to bear in mind the fact that preventive
measures, however extensive, will never eliminate adverse
effects entirely, and that the cost factor is still only one aspect
of the distress which adverse effects can involve.

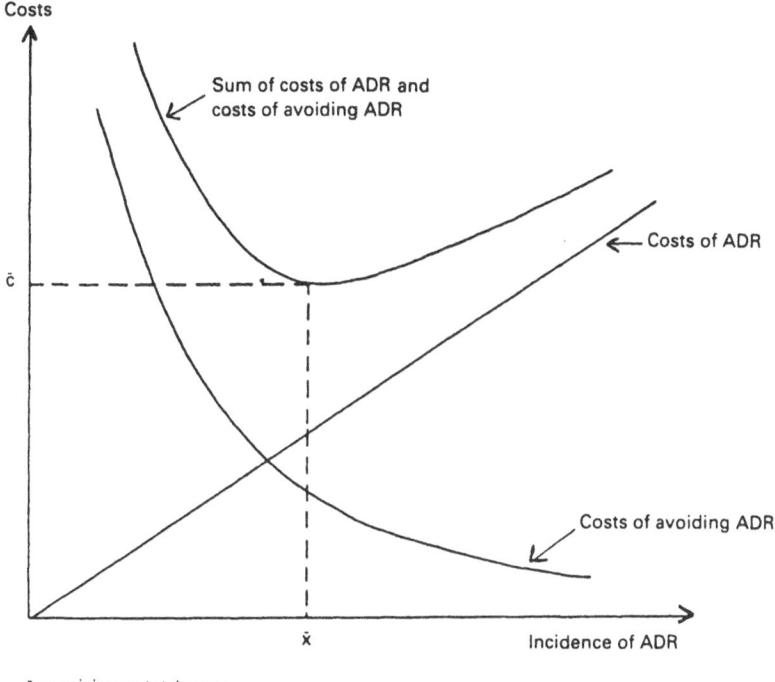

Costs

$\bar{c}$ = minimum total costs
$\hat{x}$ = optimal incidence of ADR

Figure 1 Costs of ADR and costs of avoiding ADR

Effects on research and innovation Research might be affected either negatively or positively by the policies of drug regulatory agencies. The principal concerns expressed by the drug industry are that regulation increases the time and investment needed for development, causing companies to shift from high-risk innovative research to low-risk 'me-too' activities, and emburdening research units with an unnecessarily large amount of non-creative work. Among the most pessimistic prognostications is that of Cromie[24]; writing in the United Kingdom in 1977 on regulatory repercussions he remarked that '. . . there is little to encourage anybody to invest in pharmaceutical research with the return on investment in the United Kingdom being about 6 per cent in 1974 and nearer 3 per cent in 1975 and 1976, while the average for industry remained about 10 per cent.' Certainly the traditional pathways to pharmaceutical discovery and development – the serendipity route and the repeated cycling of information from laboratory experiment to clinical observation and back – are critically dependent on tests of pharmacological activity in man. The involvement of the regulatory bodies in this process (to give permission for individual clinical studies) may slow down this all important feedback process from clinic to laboratory and back again. The net result might be not only a marked increase in time for the development of a new medicine but – more importantly – a decline in the probability that successful new compounds will be developed. CIOMS has established an expert group to identify ways to get new substances to man earlier without unnecessary risk, but there are certainly no easy solutions.

Most aspects of the interrelationship between regulation and research have been the subject of studies, largely relating to other industries; in the pharmaceutical field a lot remains to be done. Some workers have used economic measures, others measures of innovative achievement such as those discussed in Chapter 3.

In the United States, the size of the research and development budget as a percentage of sales has certainly declined in both the chemical and the pharmaceutical industries over the past twenty years. All the same, publicly available data on the size of research programmes do not suggest an overall decline in drug research. The investment adviser Saks, writing 17 years after the introduction of the Kefauver amendments to drug legislation in the United States, noted a continuing growth in research by 13 of 14 large American companies, with increases in expenditure ranging between 9% (Warner Lambert) and 33% (Syntax) between 1975 and 1977[108], though the effect of inflation has to be taken into account in interpreting these figures. He remarks that 'because of the great successes of new drugs such as Motrin, Tagamet and Clinoril, allocations for research funding are being substantially increased relative to the past.' Similar conclusions are noted by other investment analysts on both sides of the Atlantic, their conclusions being substantially more optimistic than those advanced by industry in the regulatory debate. Ashford[48] has however pointed to the fallacy of tying investment strategies all too closely to supposed effects on research. The innovative record of companies with similar investment in research can differ very greatly because of their dissimilar scientific abilities and strategies. The matter might better be studied in specific situations. An alternative approach is to look at the return on investment currently offered by new drugs, a matter which will be discussed later.

Approaching the matter at the level of successful innovation, there seems to be no gross evidence that, as measured in purely quantitative terms, the 'barren harvest' of new drugs forecast as resulting from drug regulation is developing as an overall trend at the present time. According to a survey published in December 1983[74], the number of drugs currently in research worldwide was estimated at 4209, with 2110 still in the pre-clinical phase but 675 already launched in one or more countries. The number of new chemical entities launched in 1981 amounted to 65, in 1982 to 39 and in 1983 again to 39. Once more, however, we must remind ourselves that figures like this mean very little unless we know the names of the drugs and can assess their innovative significance, e.g. on the Lunde/ Dukes scale.

Not all the effects of regulatory activity on research are necessarily negative. A high but reasonable standard of regulation is in theory likely to create fewer problems for major innovative undertakings than for the non-research based company or the less well-equipped firm; in the short run this could mean a shift of business to the former and in the long run it could lead to complete withdrawal of the latter from the field[92]; if that happened it could mean that a larger proportion of the money spent on drugs would end up in innovative research. This point could probably be studied objectively using international comparisons over a period of time.

A longer-term positive effect could be the catalysation of technological change – what Martin has termed a 'technology push'[76]. As he puts it:

> '. . . there is at least some evidence that social standards of production and economic performance of affected firms are not necessarily in conflict with each other and can even be complementary. Numerous cases have been reported in which firms have developed or adopted technological innovations enabling them to meet such standards while maintaining or even improving their economic performance, sometimes dramatically. . . . Such changes undoubtedly lie towards one end of a continuum, with firms unable to meet the standards without going bankrupt at the other end . . .'

There is certainly evidence of positive effects of regulation on other types of industry. Inspectors who visit manufacturers may sometimes act more like consultants than investigators. One study of government influences on innovation in five countries (other than the United States) found that innovations for ordinary business purposes were much more likely to be commercially successful when environmental, health and safety concerns were present as an element in the planning process than when they were absent[109]. Technological changes well beyond the scope of the compliance effort were found to have been associated with the need to comply with regulations. In delineating this phenomenon, Allen has suggested that it may arise most often in industries not previously innovative and may occur because of the necessity, brought on by regulation, to rethink established and previously unquestioned modes of operation[81]. Similarly, one does hear incidentally of constructive proposals made by regulatory officials and committees to help applicants in completing their development projects; because of their broad experience, regulatory agencies should be very well equipped to give such advice; it is not clear how often this in fact happens.

Regulation may also modify research patterns in various ways, affecting the spectrum of drugs in study; one might be tempted to attribute the relatively low proportion of truly innovative research, as identified by Offerhaus[70] to regulatory causes, thus confirming one of industry's fears on this score. The findings in the European Studies to date, though very preliminary, do not support this theory. One of the earliest European Studies, examining new drug applications in Norway and the Netherlands[69], provided an example of this. The overall acceptance rate for fully innovative drugs was 68% in the Netherlands and 79% in Norway, but the acceptance rate for semi-innovative drugs (many of them products representing the less inspired form of molecular manipulation) was only 48% and 43% respectively. Coupled with the less attractive marketing possibilities for the latter type of product, this regulatory effect could therefore markedly discourage what is sometimes called 'me-too' research, leading companies to concentrate either on high-risk high-reward innovative work or at the other extreme on the development of low-cost generic and similar products. This could in turn catalyse a further restructuring of the pharmaceutical industry.

In a comparable study from the United Kingdom[61], it was found that fully innovative products very rarely failed to pass the Committee on Safety of Medicines; only 4 of 103 negative decisions related to compounds of this type. Again in the United Kingdom, Steward & Wibberley noted that the proportion of newly marketed new chemical entities which in their view showed 'little or no advantage' over earlier drugs dropped from 32% in 1960–1963 to 18% in 1967–1970[113, 114].

Finally, effects on innovation can of course be exercised indirectly in various ways. As Steward has pointed out, '. . . general control over the output of innovation could be exerted by increasing the knowledge of consumers so that the market operates more effectively (for example by controlling advertising and providing independent information).' The type of influence which this writer has in mind clearly relates to the elimination of an unjustified demand for products of no proven value (e.g. those hallowed only by tradition) so that there is less reason for a company to seek to innovate in these areas. To date regulatory agencies have not been so active in consumer education that there is very much to investigate.

Effects on the economy   If the pharmaceutical industry is in financial difficulties, as a result of regulation or for any other reason, one would expect this to emerge from publicly available trading figures. Those which one encounters do not suggest that the gloomier prophecies as to the future of a regulated industry are being fulfilled, though it could be argued that the industry has so far succeeded in maintaining its position by diversification and by expansion in less tightly regulated markets. An overview of the world pharmaceutical industry published in December 1983[74] and covering the period 1982–1983 showed that during this period:

– the world's 15 largest pharmaceutical companies (whose percentage interest in pharmaceuticals ranged from 16.7% to 81.7%) achieved sales ranging from $1,215.5 millions to $2,628.1 million with sales increases in all cases, which ranged from 3.0% to 23.5%;

– the profit margin of the ten most profitable companies ranged from 26.74% to 49.23%;

– research and development expenditure amounted to $276.8 million at Hoechst, $184.4 million at Boehringer Ingelheim, $183.6 million at Sandoz and an estimated $463.13 million at Roche.

According to *The Times*' '1000' review of leading companies[75] the 100 largest European corporations in 1982 included 9 with substantial interests in the pharmaceutical field; the highest ranking were Hoechst at 10th place, Bayer at 12th place and Ciba-Geigy at 31st place. The corresponding list of the largest American companies includes only 2 with important interests in pharmaceuticals. It is not clear whether this difference is significant. It could simply reflect the fact that an international pharmaceutical company has to attain a certain level for efficient and productive research-based operation, and that since the average size of large American companies as a group is greater than that in Europe, pharmaceutical firms are less likely to reach the 'top hundred'. Since however virtually no large company operates exclusively in the pharmaceutical field, figures like these are only of limited interest; the main fact which they confirm, if confirmation were needed, is that large European companies still consider it very well worth while, despite a diversity of interests, to continue in the ethical pharmaceutical business.

The situation in the United States is better illustrated by examining the records of the United States Federal Trade Commission, which indicate the rate of return to shareholders in various types of industry over a certain period of time (Table VIII). Although, as Grabowski points out[91], the accounting measure used may overstate profitability for fast-growing research intensive industries (because they expend rather than capitalize investments in intangible capital such as research and development investment outlays) the pharmaceutical industry emerges as being extremely (and perhaps increasingly) profitable.

Broadly similar figures were collected in the United Kingdom in 1983 for the Parliamentary Public Accounts Committee; it is however generally difficult to compile meaningful figures of this type within Europe, where home markets are smaller and most research-based companies are multinational, taking profits and earnings in those countries where the taxation climate is most favourable. The figures on pharmaceutical profits made available to investors (rather than on the framework of the regulatory controversy) suggest however that the research-based pharmaceutical industry remains very profitable and anticipates marked growth in the years to come[93, 163] though investment advisers commonly disagree even as to the prospects for large and successful companies[127].

Since there are no gross signs of an overall decline in the pharmaceutical industry, one can hardly expect to detect a

Table VIII Rate of return on stockholder equity (net of taxes) in selected research intensive industries in the United States.

Industry	Year				
	1976	1977	1978	1979	1980*
Pharmaceuticals	18.0	18.2	18.8	19.3	20.8
Instruments	14.7	16.8	17.9	16.8	17.0
Aerospace	12.8	15.0	15.6	18.4	16.1
Electrical equipment	12.8	15.2	16.7	17.4	15.0
All manufacturing	13.9	14.2	15.0	16.4	13.9

*1980 values based on the first three quarters data.

Data compiled by Grabowski[91] from Quarterly Financial Reports 1975–1980, US Federal Trade Commission.

major adverse effect of regulation by analyses at this overall level though this leaves unanswered the crucial question as to what greater development might have occurred had there been less regulation or none at all. Once again, it proves better to turn from generalities to specific cases and try to examine the profitability of individual new drugs. Grawbowski & Vernon[93] have developed a model for determining this figure and have applied it to 37 drugs discovered in the United States during the period 1970–1976[94]. One of their conclusions was that only 13 of these 37 drugs covered both their research costs and the interest which could have been earned had this money instead been invested at current rates; they also conclude that twelve years or more of patent-protected sales are needed to provide such a return. No comparable work has been undertaken in Europe. Verifiable calculations of this type could be useful in determining whether demands for an extension of patent life should be granted, either generally or in special instances. Irrespective of whether the figures actually apply to Europe or not, they illustrate the effect which unnecessary regulatory delay may have upon the finances of a new product.

It is however clear that the prospects for profitability of a real new drug, as compared to the profitability calculated retrospectively in a historical model, is extremely difficult to predict. In retrospect it is easy to say that one could have foreseen the remarkable effects of the introduction of propranolol on the growth of ICI in the United Kingdom or of cimetidine on the turnover of Smith Kline and French in the United States[128] but at the time of their evaluation it was not at all certain how widely they would be accepted into medicine. For the second drug entering such a new field, such as ranitidine (which followed cimetidine), predictions are even more uncertain, since much will depend on the ultimate pattern of adverse effects emerging in practice, and naturally also upon the marketing approach adopted. These factors, as well as the interpretation put upon them by the stock market[128], can mean much more than any regulatory measure in determining the effect which such a drug has upon the finances of the company which develops it.

A nation's overall economy could also be affected by drug regulation in various ways, e.g. by its effects on the profitability of large companies, by affecting the incidence of adverse reactions (which as pointed out above can be measured in economic terms) and not in the last place by influencing prescribing costs and the level of drug imports. Drug regulatory decisions in Spain are thought to have contributed to the growth of the home-based pharmaceutical industry[169]. A regulatory authority could adversely affect a country's export position by seeking to regulate drugs intended for foreign markets; at present, such regulation is, rightly or wrongly, largely limited to questions of manufacture in approved plants. On all these points claims and allegations have been made but as yet there does not seem to have been any overall study of the effect of drug regulation on any country's economy.

2. COMPARATIVE EVALUATION AND THE CONCEPT OF NEED

If a regulatory agency is authorized to reject new drugs for which there is considered to be no medical need (even if they are efficacious and safe) this is likely to have marked repercussions on the drug industry. There is fairly broad agreement among clinical pharmacologists that very few new drugs really represent an advance in therapy[70]; if the need element were to be strictly applied as part of evaluation, this could therefore result in a decimation in the flow of new products entering the market. The concept of need assessment is vigorously opposed by the pharmaceutical industry[117], mainly with the argument that medical need is difficult to assess (since the specific usefulness of a new drug may only emerge in practice) and that agencies should not unnecessarily limit the physician's choice of drugs. Less prominent, but perhaps much more realistic, is the argument that many pharmaceutical companies only contrive to grow and prosper during the long periods between major innovations by introducing less exciting products which cannot strictly be regarded as medically necessary. The need concept is only specifically incorporated in the law in a very few West European countries, notably Norway[12], where the number of drugs marketed has been kept at a low level, largely in this way. The need concept is also regularly employed in Iceland; Kristinsdottir found that of 42 drug rejections in 1981, 7 were based on the fact that no benefits had been proven[118]. However, the divorce between this Nordic approach and that of other countries is not as absolute as it seems at first sight.

Lunde & Dukes[69], comparing regulatory practice in the Netherlands and Norway, noted a striking parallel in rejection rates in the two countries despite the absence of a need clause in the Netherlands. They found that in the Norwegian situation lack of need is commonly a direct consequence of lack of merit or lack of proven safety; whether need or efficacy and safety are the considerations formally involved in taking a negative decision is a question of convenience, legal tradition and semantics rather than an expression of an absolute difference in approach. Dukes[102] has suggested that some countries without a need clause do in fact take the relative merits of a product into account, and that the mere fact that a product is a little better than a placebo will not suffice to obtain registration if it falls far short of the standard of efficacy and safety currently regarded as normal for this class of drugs. Data from Granat *et al.*[64] appear to confirm that this indeed happens in practice. It is also clear that a need clause in effect exists in certain countries with a centralized economy where a limited drug list is maintained and some drugs which have been accepted scientifically will not be imported because foreign exchange considerations render a further selection necessary. Exactly the same applies in many importing and developing countries where lists of essential drugs are maintained, at least for official purchasing[135].

As pointed out earlier, one practical repercussion of such need assessment policies in any shape or form is clearly to render the development of semi-innovative ('me-too') products still less attractive and thereby possibly to provide more encouragement and funding for truly innovative high-risk research; it would seem important to find out whether or not this actually happens.

3. ANIMAL STUDIES AND LONG-TERM STUDIES IN MAN

The increase over the past ten years in safety evaluation testing is a contributory factor in the rising costs of new drug development. It has been estimated that the proportion of a United Kingdom company's research and development budget allocated to pre-clinical toxicity testing has increased from 8–10% to 14–16% over the past ten years[165]. The numbers of animals required for acute, chronic, reproductive and carcinogenicity tests before a new chemical entity is used long-term in man have increased dramatically. In the early 1960's fewer than 1,000 animals were used in safety evaluation studies for a single drug; today this figure has increased threefold[166].

Whether or not this volume of work is justified is, as pointed out earlier, a matter of serious dispute. On the one hand there is pressure to undertake every form of investigation which might reduce the risk of a new drug for man; on the other there is concern that many animals are being sacrificed and large sums expended on work of limited and sometimes negligible predictive value. No simple solution to this dilemma seems likely to emerge in the near future, though tissue culture work and other techniques not using whole animals help to reduce both costs and animal usage. Some of the lack of logic in the present situation emerges from the considerable differences in animal testing requirements from agency to agency. Currently repeated dose animal toxicity studies in two species lasting 6 months are required by EEC countries for drugs marketed for long-term use in man; 12-month studies are required in the United States and 18-month studies in Canada.

Writing in 1978, Cromie pointed to the gradual accumulation of regulatory requirements as time progressed, despite the fact that the development of a new test should often make it possible to abandon an older one. 'Unfortunately' he adds, 'I do not know of a single significant reduction; all that has happened is that more and more tests have been added'[24]. Broadly speaking, Cromie was quite right; in a situation of doubt and dispute, there has been a lot of public, political and legal pressure to maintain any requirement which could conceivably help to ensure drug safety in man. What has happened, and what was already happening in 1978, is that drug regulatory agencies have banded together with others to review the situation carefully, with the result that unfavourable animal findings alone are less likely to bar a drug's path to the market. The classic instance was that of carcinogenicity testing of oral contraceptives in beagle dogs. In 1974, after the discovery of breast tumours in beagles used in such tests had already put paid to the career of megestrol and chlormadinone as oral contraceptives and was threatening to do the same for lynestrenol, Prof. Eric Scowan of Britain's Committee on Safety of Medicines convened an international meeting of regulators and investigators to review the issue. A turning point was undoubtedly the presentation of evidence that even natural progesterone, tested under the same conditions, induced mammary tumours in the beagle. The upshot of this meeting was that, although beagle testing was not abandoned, the interpretation put upon the findings was thereafter much more cautious and the study of alternative models was intensified. Since then, other initiatives have been undertaken, from quite different directions, to study impartially the value or lack of value of specific test routines, both in animals and man.

The LD_{50} acute toxicity study in animals has been heavily criticized for its lack of relevance to human safety[60]. Zbinden & Flury-Roversi, in particular, have shown that for the prediction of human lethal dose, and for the characterization of clinical toxicology, it is of limited use[62].

The scientific justification for animal toxicity studies lasting more than 6 months can be questioned as a result of preliminary work performed by Walker *et al.*[137]. Nineteen pharmaceutical companies in Europe provided comprehensive data on repeated dose animal studies of varying duration for 136 compounds studied in one or more animal species[167]. In these studies the salient effects were identified and described together with their time of occurrence, the number of animals affected and the dose. These data allow appropriate analyses to be carried out with respect to determining the predictive value of 12-, 18- or 24-month studies compared with those of up to 6 months' duration. The establishment of a computer-based toxicology data bank, by the Centre for Medicines Research in the United Kingdom, is a move towards determining the value of the animal data, if any, obtained during longer-term studies, and to explore the discrepancies between the regulatory requirements of different countries.

McNamara[176], surveying the evidence on long-term animal work, goes even further than Walker, and finds good evidence that satisfactory long-term dose levels can be established by toxicity tests of about 4 months' duration. Heywood[60] too has studied in great detail current evidence on the relevance of animal drug studies to man, including both acute and chronic toxicity data and reproduction studies. With respect to chronic studies he considers it 'generally accepted by most toxicologists that there is little information to be gained from continuing animal studies beyond six months'. A more general lesson which can be distilled from Heywood's work is the need to allow toxicity testing to evolve as new evidence on valid techniques becomes available and to adapt the tests used to the characteristics of the compound under study. It would be unfortunate if the introduction of specific toxicity requirements into regulatory guidelines, such as is happening in the European Community, were to render such adaptation more difficult.

Indirect evidence of the relatively restricted value of some animal data also emerged from the Australian study in the European series. Of 32 restrictive decisions which in retrospect proved to be justified, 31 were taken exclusively or in part on the basis of clinical data, with animal data providing supporting evidence in only 4 cases. Animal data underlay 5 of 6 marginally correct decisions, but none of the problems predicted proved to be of real clinical importance. Finally, animal studies were the main basis for 17 restrictive decisions the correctness of which could not be assessed; most of these reflected concerns as to long-term effects seen in toxicity work which several years later had been neither confirmed nor refuted in man[53].

Current doubts as to the value of long-term animal studies relate primarily to general toxicity testing. There is more agreement that in the present state of knowledge testing for carcinogenicity can with some specific exceptions (e.g. breast tumours in beagle dogs) provide evidence of value, especially when there are positive findings in both these and mutagenicity studies[59]. Teratogenicity studies, on the other hand, remain highly unsatisfactory, though there are pointers as to the way they might be improved[83].

Very similar doubts are now arising as to the need for certain types of long-term experiment in man. The Finnish regulator Idänpään-Heikkilä[26], using the internal material of the United States FDA, has produced a masterly analysis of the value of various study designs in obtaining information on adverse drug reactions. Short-term phase III trials were usually found to uncover the most frequent and acute adverse drug reactions, whilst controlled trials (against placebo or active drug) demonstrated the actual incidence of these reactions. An increase in the number of patients taking part in short-term studies from a few hundred to one thousand or more was seldom found to help in detecting rare or sporadic (but still clinically important) reactions; for both scientific and organization reasons it proved more efficient to extend short-term studies in a smaller group to 3 months rather than to treat a larger group for 1 month. Studies lasting up to 6 months, conducted with 9 products, detected fairly important adverse reactions to 2 of these which had not been found at 3 months; studies of this duration were thus valuable but did not need to be conducted under controlled conditions. Use of the life table method allowed a greater amount of clinically relevant information to be obtained from a given trial. If further work confirms these conclusions, there would seem to be very little point in studying drugs in humans for more than 6 months prior to marketing, except where the characteristics of the drug or the disease (e.g. seasonal fluctuation) suggest that this is necessary; longer-term pre-registration studies could be replaced by obligatory post-marketing investigations.

Using published material, one can also approach the question of the cost/value ratio in large-scale clinical trials from a non-regulatory point of view. Levy & Sondik[129] of the National Heart, Lung and Blood Institute in the United States have critically examined in this way the Coronary Drug Project, the Hypertension Detection and Follow-up Program and a proposed trial of anti-arrhythmic agents in the prevention of sudden death. Their methods were chosen mainly to help national health authorities in taking decisions on requests for financial support, but they would be equally applicable to certain studies likely to be required by regulatory authorities, e.g. for lipid-lowering drugs claimed to provide long-term benefits. 'Large scale clinical trials' they conclude 'are most certainly worth the cost, but only after careful deliberation and consideration of their potential impact and feasibility and an assessment of the lost opportunities that might derive from shifting funds from basic research into validation'.

A particular thorn in the flesh of the drug industry has been the requirement that certain types of work be repeated from one country to another in order to secure registration. Except in certain unusual situations, e.g. where one is dealing with a very different population or environment or where an agency has reason to believe that foreign material may not have been obtained in a bona fide manner, the requirement that scientific work be repeated nationally has fortunately become far less common in recent years. Even in the past, such requirements may not have been applied as stringently as their formulation suggests. It has for example often been stated that 'prior to 1975 the FDA did not accept foreign data at all as positive evidence'[91] and indeed in the cromolyn study[71], the FDA, unlike the other European agencies studied, was found to have required national clinical work; material from foreign studies was however fully evaluated and played a role in the approval.

There does not seem to be any justification for repeating valid preclinical pharmacology from country to country; French and Japanese rats are likely to be biologically identical[36].

4. THE EFFICIENCY OF REGULATION

Whether an agency is efficient or not is a question which can partially – but only partially – be answered by examining the time taken to deal with specific matters. Efficiency or inefficiency can also be reflected in such matters as the quality of the decisions, the openness of communications with applicants, and the extent to which matters raised by the agency relate to truly relevant medical and scientific issues or to mere formalities.

Time taken to deal with applications   The principal accusations of delay have been directed at the United States FDA[79]. For example, in one study of the work of the FDA[26], the total processing time for three psychopharmacological drugs was 61.4 months. About half this time was used by companies to provide amendments as a response to FDA action letters. Of a mean new drug development time of about 8.2 years, about 3.9 years was used for phase I and phase II trials and only 1.8 years for the phase III trials. The mean processing time for new drug applications from submission to approval/non-approval was about 2.4 years – or 30% of the total time for new drug development.

A number of European countries, such as Sweden[13,175] have been regarded as unduly slow in the processing of applications, others have not. In the initial comparison of Netherlands and Norwegian practice in the European series, Lunde & Dukes[69] found that applications accepted in less than 12 months comprised 93 of 225 in the former country and 87 of 213 in the latter; the great bulk of decisions were taken in less than 18 months. In the cromolyn sodium study in the European series[71] the registration time between five countries varied from 10 to 42.5 months, though this was in part due to disputed evidence from safety studies which became available whilst certain agencies were still dealing with the application; the 10–12.5 month approval period attained by three agencies, despite the fact that the product was novel as regards its structure, form of application and mode of action, could be regarded as very favourable.

However, even relatively efficient agencies can experience difficult periods if their capacity is marginal; ten Ham[130], in the Netherlands, found that the 'RD 90' (maximum duration of registration for 90% of applications) rose from about 23 months in 1971 to about 37 months in 1976 and then fell again to about 28 months in 1980. It was notable that the increase in registration time, though not correlated with the number of applications received yearly, occurred at a time when an additional strain was being placed on the agency's resources by the existence of the joint Benelux regulatory procedure. Similarly in Iceland[118] Kristinsdottir, noted an average handling time which increased progressively from 11.1 months in 1977 to 18.4 months in 1981, with a range from 1 month to 44 months.

In their five-country comparison, covering the period 1960–1961. Hass *et al.*[78] measured the lag occurring between the first introduction of a new chemical entity in any one of the five countries (France, the Federal Republic of Germany, Italy, the United Kingdom and the United States) and its introduction, if ever, in the others. They found that the average lag for original molecules available in the countries with the shortest lag times was about two years. France, the Federal Republic of Germany and the United Kingdom were operating at about this rate for molecules first introduced on the five-country market between 1963 and 1972. In the United States the average lag was about 1.7 years for molecules first introduced on the five-country market in 1960. By the end of the decade, the average American lag had increased to about four years, but returned to about 2.25 years for molecules first introduced on the five-country market in the early 1970s. Writing in March 1982, they note that 'the average lag for original molecules introduced on the five-country market cannot be precisely determined for recent years at this time. However, the percentage of original molecules introduced on a single country market during their first year of availability has been a good barometer (inversely related) of the lag for all molecules eventually introduced. This percentage for the U.S.A. was lowest in the late 1960s (around 10 per cent). During the 1970s this percentage has varied between 11 and 14. Currently it is about 14 per cent, indicating that the eventual lag for 1979–1981 will be relatively low. Similar arguments indicate that lag times for France increased in the mid 1970's but are currently on a continuous decline. In Italy lag time decreased steadily from 1964 through 1978 but have increased significantly over the last two years. In the U.K. lag times have increased significantly since 1976.'

The Hass study, undertaken by FDA staff, provides clear confirmation of earlier work by others on the so-called drug lag in the United States. However, as they point out, every country has a drug lag if one compares the date of introduction of new chemical entities with their first introductions elsewhere, and the casual or unsophisticated observer in each of the five countries could conclude that 'new drugs are introduced more slowly in my country than in the other countries'.

A number of other methodological points arise from this work. One has to bear in mind that the term drug lag is not always used in the same sense in the literature. Sometimes it refers to the absolute non-availability of certain drugs in some countries (generally because they are refused); or it can refer to the delay in taking positive decisions; or it can relate to the lateness of new drug introductions, which are sometimes caused by late submission of the application in a particular country rather than by agency delay. In the first sense, Norway and Iceland have a very pronounced drug lag but their procedures are not on average exceptionally slow. The Hass study does not go into the question as to whether drugs which never became available in certain markets were in fact useful and necessary, nor does it look at the question of priorities in dealing with new drug applications. Where an agency has too little capacity to deal with all applications promptly it may, either systematically or by instinct, choose to deal first with those applications which relate to therapeutic innovations. Whether this selection is carried out in a fair and open manner or not is a point which needs to be examined.

Communication with applicants The more willing an agency is to discuss problems with an applicant across the table, the less the risk of misunderstanding and delay. In a few countries, such as the Netherlands, an applicant has a legal right to a hearing if the agency raises any objection at all to the registration of a product, and in many other countries hearings have become customary because both parties find them useful. In the European study of the cromolyn sodium application[71], hearings with the manufacturer were held in four of the five countries and proved mutually beneficial; only in Norway was the contact with the agency minimal.

There also seems to be a need for open communication on a

broader level. Regular contact meetings and the publication of guidelines to help companies in preparing applications and understanding agency policies are more usual in some countries than others, yet they appear to facilitate the regulatory process by eliminating misunderstandings. Klaes *et al.*, looking at the philosophies of various regulatory agencies, have expressed the view, though without documenting it fully, that some agencies become isolated from the world which they are supposed to regulate; these authors believe that there is a correlation between such isolation and what they call a 'high intensity of regulation'[66]. It is clear, however, that such contacts may, unless they are sufficiently open, be viewed by the outside world as evidence of connivance between agencies and industry, providing an opportunity for the latter to exert undue influence[123]. If these suspicions are to be allayed, it may be important to allow for other parties, such as representatives of patients and consumers, to meet with an agency on matters of public importance. Most countries have no provision for such contacts.

Realistic or unrealistic objections   At its worst, an agency (and perhaps particularly one which has become isolated from the real world, as described above) can lay greater weight on the exact letter of the law than on a medically relevant interpretation of the problems facing it. The Norwegian/Dutch comparison in the European series shows that in studying this question one has to distinguish between formal ('overcomable') objections to registration which almost always arise in the early stages of any application, and those which are essential, absolute and lead an application to be rejected or substantially modified. The former can lead to delays but the latter are of the greatest interest in studying an agency's policies, and determining how realistic they are. In that study it was found that of 149 essential objections to 100 rejected applications in the Netherlands, 92 related to clinical efficacy and 41 to clinical safety. Only 10 essential objections were raised on grounds of animal pharmacology or toxicology, and 6 on pharmaceutical grounds, and most of these occurred in parallel with clinical objections. This would suggest a realistic approach to applications. The findings in Norway were similar, except for the influence of the 'need paragraph', the effects of which have already been discussed. The finding in this and other studies (e.g. that on non-steroidal anti-inflammatory agents[50]) that two agencies working entirely independently of each other can take quite similar decisions and achieve a similar acceptance rate again suggests that objections are reasonably realistic. Data from the United Kingdom on grounds for acceptance or rejection are fairly comparable. Griffin & Diggle[61] noted in a series of 103 applications withdrawn after notification of pending rejection that safety had featured as a ground for the Committee's concern in 75.8% of these applications, efficacy in 69.1% and quality in only 30.0%.

In this connection one can also study the extent to which the practice of a national agency is in tune with informed medical opinion as reflected in the literature. Buurma *et al.*[68], examining the policies of the Netherlands Committee in the light of current medical opinion found a 'large measure of agreement between the view of the Committee and pharmacotherapeutic views emerging from subsequent practice.'

Problems involving more than one evaluation discipline (e.g. both pharmacy and pharmacology) From isolated experiences one can conclude that there is a risk in regulatory procedures of a single discipline advancing objections (e.g. pharmaceutical or toxicological) which in the light of the clinical assessment prove to be irrelevant or overridden. These may nevertheless be maintained unless there is a procedure for joint and mutual assessment of the entire file, e.g. by a committee. The cromolyn study[71] threw light on such problems; they appeared however to be dealt with efficiently by all agencies where they arose.

Efficiency of appeal procedures It is a basic tenet of administrative law that there must be a right of appeal from the decisions of an official body; such procedures exist in most countries. In principle both scientific and administrative matters should be open to appeal. However, the channels of appeal may not be adequate or may not function sufficiently. In Norway, for example, the applicant can apply for scientific reconsideration of the case but only to the same body which took the original decision. In the Netherlands, some evidence published by ten Ham indicates that the appeal procedure may be very slow, thus undermining the right of a new drug applicant to a fair hearing or the ability of the agency to remove an ineffective or unsafe product from the market. 'A problem is that for "old" products a negative decision by the Agency will not be effectuated if the applicant appeals to the Crown. This means that the product can remain on the market until the Crown, after consulting the Council of State, gives its judgement on appeal. The latter unfortunately can be delayed. A well known example is that of Vasolastine. In 1966 registration of this product was refused. The manufacturer appealed and not until 1978 was judgement passed down, which confirmed the Agency's decision. Until that time the product was able to remain on the market.'[130]

5

Conclusions and recommendations

1. OVERALL IMPRESSIONS TO DATE

The experience gained with the basic approaches outlined in Chapter 2 is still limited, but most of them seem to be valid and useful provided they are employed impartially and conscientiously.

The evidence available to date does not, in any country, enable one to measure adequately the total effect of the drug regulatory system in force. Some of the methods available are unsatisfactory and even where techniques have been devised relatively little work has been undertaken. This is not a shortcoming which relates to the drug field alone; in most areas of public health too little is known about the effects of legislation and regulation and the means to measure them. What existing work does do is to disprove or throw doubt on some of the more extreme views which have been expressed about drug regulation in the course of the years. Some such lessons may be briefly stated.

Firstly, there is no reasonable doubt that *drug regulatory agencies play an essential role in defending the public interest.* The mere existence of an agency maintaining high standards may of itself be enough to discourage applications for the marketing of ineffective, unsafe or unproven products; the proportion of drugs rejected is in countries with experienced agencies very high and there are important parallels between such negative decisions. For such reasons, self-regulation by individual pharmaceutical companies, the standards of which vary markedly, would not always provide adequate protection for the public. These conclusions apply primarily to questions of efficacy and safety. So far in Europe matters of quality control have provoked less interest but the matter requires further study.

Secondly, however, even where the broad policies of agencies run parallel, there can be substantial *differences of detail in their decisions*. Approved indications, contraindications, and warnings differ considerably and they probably have only a limited influence on patterns of medical prescribing.

Thirdly, regulation has *not succeeded in preventing a succession of serious drug problems* leading to the withdrawal of new products shortly after their introduction. A careful retrospective study of these cases might indicate how modified regulatory systems could protect the public more completely from such incidents.

Fourthly, it is not generally true that regulatory agencies have a large backlog of applications relating to products representing *major therapeutic advances*. Formally or informally, the agencies the records of which have so far been amenable to study seem to be able to ensure that, even where there is an accumulation of unfinished work, the (apparently very few) products which represent real breakthroughs will be dealt with promptly and efficiently. The concept of the drug lag, which was developed primarily with respect to delays in approval in the United States, and which has been a variable phenomenon even there, must not blindly be applied to agencies elsewhere.

Fifthly, however, even efficient agencies do on occasion suffer periods of overloading or understaffing, during which a backlog of work arises. Every agency so far examined appears to have a major problem in that its *capacity is at times insufficient* to deal promptly with the entire programme of work. This means that, even though special measures may be taken to avoid impeding major therapeutic advances, manufacturers may find their normal course of business seriously hindered by the time needed to obtain approval of new formulations or modified claims. Since the costs of regulation are negligible with respect to those of drug development, substantially higher fees for regulatory applications might where necessary be set in order to ensure that agencies can retain adequate and experienced staff.

Even where incoming work is dealt with efficiently, it is clear that most or all agencies have little capacity available for such general matters as the development of consistent policies and the updating of older decisions; many data sheets in use for drugs on the market are out of date, and where a manufacturer does not request the agency for permission to update them the latter will rarely itself take the initiative except when an acute situation arises. Factors such as these clearly impair the influence of an agency.

Sixthly, there are still very marked *differences* from country to country between the range of activities subject to regulatory control and the extent to which allowance is made for traditional national patterns of medical behaviour and prescribing. The former type of discrepancy might be reduced by an objective study of priorities – one might for example examine the hypothesis that in Western Europe there is much more need to regulate advertising than quality standards. The latter type of discrepancy seems likely to decline spontaneously as time passes since the true interests of public health do not differ greatly from country to country.

Lastly, drug regulation has clearly affected the *pattern of research* in the drug industry. It is one of the factors which has raised the costs of drug development but there is no conclusive evidence of a deterious effect on the flow of truly innovative new products. However, unreasonable requirements have sometimes been set and industry believes that many agencies are slow to modify, redraft, and reformulate their requirements in the light of changes in knowledge. Such objections need to be taken seriously and these faults remedied.

2. TECHNIQUES FOR FURTHER STUDIES

Future studies of drug regulation should obviously in the first place comprise an extension of what has already been done successfully. Existing work relates only to a few agencies, companies and products and to a limited time period; it provides useful impressions but there is a lot that needs to be confirmed. Continuing the present type of work for a longer period will also throw light on the sometimes considerable fluctuations in the performance of all the parties concerned.

In addition, however, there is plenty of scope for using new methods, including some which have been tested in other fields of regulation. Certain of these methods may be sketched here.

Prospective studies Although in many respects, as pointed out earlier, the medical literature will ultimately provide a reliable verdict on the effects of regulation, a clearer view is likely to be obtained by prospective studies; these could be undertaken, for example, when a new class of drugs is introduced for the first time (e.g. as happened in the case of the first H–2 blocker), and especially where regulatory policies with respect to these drugs differ from country to country.

Some five to seven years of concerted effort may be needed before the effects of a regulatory measure can be properly judged, in view of the long-term repercussions which it may have. Such long-term studies should preferably be conducted with the full cooperation of the pharmaceutical industry, which can supply documented evidence not otherwise available.

Studies of the quality of decisions Studies of the quality of decisions of individual agencies are needed to determine whether in retrospect they have been in keeping with the development of medicine. Here a degree of subjectivity is hard to avoid and it will be preferable to analyse practice over a long period of time after medical and scientific opinion on the issues in question has clearly crystallized out. One may have to study certain matters by collating opinions rather than by exact analysis, e.g. when assessing the extent to which a regulatory body has indeed sensed and aided the development of a broad social consensus on some matter.

In principle it should also be possible to estimate the consequences of the acceptance or retention of ineffective drugs as a result of inadequate regulatory supervision in a particular country. This could be done both in health terms and broadly also in economic terms (cost to the health service of useless therapeutic agents, but also employment provided by their production).

Retrospective studies of drug accidents Some individual instances in which newly marketed drugs have been withdrawn because of serious adverse effects[70] deserve to be investigated objectively once the emotions have calmed down and legal actions have been settled. Such work could throw light on the reasons why these problems were not anticipated at the time of registration; more realistic approaches to pre-marketing regulatory requirements might result[123].

Policies with respect to drugs claiming long-term benefits Certain types of drug are claimed primarily to offer very long-term prophylactic or other benefits. Typical is the case of lipid-lowering drugs which are intended to reduce the risk of development of atherosclerosis. There appears to be no clear and agreed policy as to the standards which the community should set for the admission of these drugs to the market. Short-term studies, reasonably feasible for the individual manufacturer when taking into account both the expenses involved and the duration of patent protection, will demonstrate only the acute pharmacodynamic properties of the drug, leaving the long-term significance of these effects entirely unsettled. This is an instance where the establishment of realistic pre-marketing requirements might block creative and much-needed research. A collaborative study of existing approaches to these problems and their effects upon research programmes could supply the basis for a constructive solution.

'Paired' studies It would be instructive to examine the differences in both the application and the regulatory proceedings between a drug which has been promptly approved and has proven commercially successful and another of a similar type which has either been rejected entirely or the commercial failure of which has been blamed on regulatory intransigence or delay. This could throw useful light on the effects of regulatory assessment on the company and its research in these contrasting cases but also on the extent to which in these contrasting conditions assessments are realistic and applications are reasonably adequate.

Comparative studies to determine the practical effect of legal provisions for the 'conditional' release of new drugs. Most countries do not have this possibility, and the pharmaceutical industry has generally considered that release of a new drug should be unconditional, except for approval of the data sheet. It has however been argued that if drugs could be released conditionally, e.g. with restrictions as regards distribution or promotion, certain problematical but useful compounds might become available earlier, e.g. to specialists, than is currently the case. The cromolyn sodium study in the European series[71] noted for example that Norway was the only one of the five countries studied to impose conditions, releasing the drug initially only for use by specialists in internal medicine and by chest physicians. It appeared that if restricted release had not been possible under Norwegian law, the drug would not have been released at all at the early stage, and that asthmatics might have been deprived of it for a further two years at least.

One regulatory approach favoured by the pharmaceutical industry is to release new compounds more readily but to intensify post-marketing surveillance and adverse drug reaction monitoring[117,121]. Cost/benefit studies of such an approach, where it has been adopted, should be carried out, preferably prospectively. Effective post-marketing surveillance is an extremely costly operation and one needs to know for what type of drugs (e.g. major innovations) such a shift in regulatory policy can be justified both in terms of expense and of risk to the public.

Study of contacts between agencies and the industry The need for such contacts has been set out in an earlier section, but so too have the accusations of 'connivance' between agencies and manufacturers. Lesser has written of such contact:

'It is probably best regarded as a . . . way of enabling two parties, representing different, occasionally even conflicting interests, to rub along together without too much friction. Practolol and benoxaprofen show, however, that such a cosy partnership not only cannot stand the strain of a disaster, but also leads to a complete paralysis of action in the resultant crisis. CSM [Committee on Safety of Medicines] fears to take the first step that might disrupt its partnership with industry . . .'[123]

Communication has sometimes been rendered more difficult by the fact that some companies and agencies have appointed professional negotiating staff so that scientists no longer speak directly to scientists. Concerns such as these can be examined by comparing the way in which various agencies handle their contacts with the pharmaceutical industry, both routinely and in situations of crisis.

Studies of other regulatory activities Studies of regulatory activities to date have been concentrated largely on the approval of new compounds. Analogous studies could be envisaged for most or all of the regulatory activities listed in Table IV in the countries where these matters are subject to control (e.g. drug distribution and advertising). Studies of the influence of regulatory bodies on prescribing practice[52] need in particular to be extended; while it is not intended that the prescriber should himself be regulated, it is of concern if prescribers use drugs in a manner which impartial and expert opinion has concluded is improper or unsafe without being aware of these authoritative opinions. Similarly, the dissemination of adverse reaction data by official bodies needs to be critically examined; work by Griffin & D'Arcy suggests that in this respect there is a lot of room for improvement[58]. Finally, it is important to determine whether measures designed to provide the prescriber with essential information are in fact being put into effect in a realistic manner; if warnings are unclear or are made available by a manufacturer only in small and scarcely legible print[150] they will have no effect at all.

Studies of the adaptability of regulatory procedures New research developments can confront agencies with problems not anticipated by the legislature, but which have to be settled in the spirit of the law. There are a number of instances where this has happened and a study of the way in which such matters have been dealt with could indicate how they can be handled intelligently and in the public interest. Typical is the emergence of recombinant DNA technology as a means of synthesizing drugs. As Bristow & Bangham wrote of this specific issue: 'It will be up to control authorities to help ensure the safety of the patient whilst providing a framework in which full advantage can be taken of this challenging and exciting breakthrough in drug therapy.[131]

Studies of the effects of regulation on self-medication Self-medication, using either drugs expressly intended for lay treatment or products intended primarily for the physician's use but in some countries readily available without prescription, is a chapter apart. Self-medication has persisted and developed on a large scale despite the availability of low-cost medical and pharmaceutical services. It is clearly necessary to determine not only the effects of regulations concerned directly with self-medication but also the extent to which regulations affecting prescription drugs result in a shift of drug usage into or out of the self-medication field. An investigation of the current scope and pattern of self-medication in Europe, initiated in 1982 by the World Health Organization, could provide useful starting material for such studies.

Studies of regulatory staffing and procedures There is already much hard evidence that some drug regulatory agencies are grossly understaffed. It is particularly disturbing to see evidence advanced that even in a large agency the overburdening of a single individual can disrupt the entire process of new drug approval[107,147]. Of equal concern is the fact that experienced drug regulators, capable of representing the public interest well, have so often been induced to accept senior positions with the pharmaceutical industry, apparently at substantially higher salaries[154].

Just as important is the general quality of staffing; from interviews one cannot avoid the impression that the pharmaceutical industry sometimes finds itself confronted with assessors or other regulatory staff who are only marginally capable of performing their task and may have no adequate insight into all the problems involved.

Study of confidentiality clauses Currently, these clauses can impede both adoption of common approaches and the performance of studies. One should determine how they should be formulated, and how they ought to be interpreted. One might also try to determine whether confidentiality clauses lead to increased costs or increase the time taken to deal with applications.

Study of pharmaceutical control performed by agencies
Some agencies perform pharmaceutical laboratory control of new drugs before they are approved, whilst other countries rely upon post-marketing analysis of random samples from pharmacies. Pre-approval verification of pharmaceutical data in the laboratory is an expensive procedure and it would seem important, in those countries where it is carried out, to determine its cost/benefit ratio.

Study of the effects of internationalization   The trend to regional drug control, as exemplified by legislation within the European Community, has developed mainly for economic reasons; if there is to be free movement of goods and services between member states, common standards for products have to be set. With the Benelux experience in mind, it will be of great importance to follow developments in the Community carefully in order to determine to what extent they do affect public health, research and the economy either beneficially or adversely.

Study of the value of 'me-too' drugs   Semi-innovative ('me-too') products are those that offer little or no advantage over existing drugs within the same therapeutic group. Many countries would like to reduce their number and some have done so drastically. By doing so one might however, as the pharmaceutical industry has so often argued, run the risk of rejecting products that later could prove to offer some unanticipated benefits. It would therefore be of interest to study the history of such products within different therapeutic classes (e.g. beta-blockers, non-steroidal anti-inflammatory drugs) over a period, to see whether their known indications and adverse reactions change and whether such products do ultimately serve the public interest or merely result in new risks and higher costs.

This list of methods and matters which might be considered in future studies is certainly not complete; the essential point will surely be to put to the test all those hypotheses which point to possible shortcomings in current regulatory systems and prospects for their improvement.

3. THE CONCEPT OF AN INTEGRATED DRUGS POLICY

One common failing appears to exist in all those countries where regulatory practice has been examined to date; nowhere does an attempt seem to have been made to develop a total drugs policy which would take into account all the elements – ranging from efficacy and safety to the impact on investment and research – discussed in this review. In most countries, indeed, the assessment of these matters, insofar as they are regulated at all, is entrusted to various unassociated bodies (e.g. drugs committees, health funds and departments of economic affairs) with no proper provision for an integration of their activities. The consequences which this could have are evident. A drugs committee composed entirely of scientists may find itself, when proposing to reject a drug on grounds of unproven (though probable) efficacy, confronted with arguments as to the repercussions on employment which it is neither technically nor legally competent to consider. Again, a pricing committee may develop policies which are relatively favourable to companies not engaged in research. A health insurance or reimbursement system may similarly favour a low-priced product rather than one the turnover of which may contribute to a major research programme, since research is not its concern[126]. To carry this last example a stage further: a body favouring a more expensive drug because of its potential contribution to research funding would probably not be legally competent to seek an undertaking that the funds earned from a higher price would indeed accrue to research rather than to advertising or company profits[134]. Again, if a drug is of such a nature that it is likely to be misused by a small minority of the population, one may have to weigh this risk against its value for others; nevertheless at the present day the official bodies dealing with drug misuse are sometimes quite different from those dealing with efficacy and safety. It is not the present argument that all the above matters need be regulated, but it is a fact that they currently are regulated in many countries, and where this is the case they should surely be dealt with in a coordinated manner as part of a total policy designed to serve the community's interests best.

If an integrated policy on drugs is to be developed, its ultimate purposes will have to be defined. The purposes of social regulation, of which drug regulation forms part, are viewed differently by economists, social theorists and those concerned with technology[105]. Environmental, health and safety regulation, as seen by economists, has as its purpose the correction of market imperfections in order to internalize the social costs of industrial production. The social theorist not only focuses on the distributive costs of regulation, but in some cases also sees regulation serving a redistributive function between the regulated industry and the intended beneficiaries of regulation, such as workers, consumers and the general public; questions of justice and fairness drive the decision-making process. Technologists will be concerned with the effects of regulation on the use and development of technology. An integrated drugs policy will need to take all these different approaches into account at the levels of legislation, regulation and day-to-day interpretation.

4. THE NEED FOR A SCIENTIFIC BASIS FOR POLICY

At the present day, much effort is made to ensure that government policies in various fields are based on a scientific (and particularly an economically defensible) approach. In the area of health, the fact that one is dealing largely with an imponderable ('good health') the measurement of which in financial terms is likely to be somewhat artificial, complicates the issue[174]. The rapid and spasmodic growth of drug regulation may also have weighed against a methodical approach; other hindrances seem to have been the dogmatic nature of much medical belief and the heavy lobbying, particularly by the pharmaceutical industry in what it regarded as its own best interests. There is today no reason why some better approach to policy making should not be undertaken, whatever the practical problems. Such work should indicate on the one hand whether an agency is attaining the ideals set for it, and on the other hand whether these ideals are, in the light of current knowledge, so ideal after all.

There would naturally be little point in conducting studies on drug regulation procedures and their effects unless the knowledge gained were indeed to be used to change practice. It seems very likely, however, that proper investigation in this field will have such an effect, and several examples are to hand to confirm this. Griffin & D'Arcy's[58] study in 1981 of the information lag showed that there was much room for improvement in the dissemination of information by drug regulatory authorities to the medical profession on adverse reactions; this led to a change of practice in the United Kingdom and Twomey & Griffin[158] were able to report in 1983 that the situation had improved considerably. Again, after Griffin & Diggle[61] recorded a dramatic fall in the number of clinical trials being conducted in the United Kingdom over the period 1971–1981 from 170 to 87 per annum, this finding led to a change in the regulations which was designed to stimulate clinical drug research and resulted in an increase in the number of clinical trial applications granted to 207 in the first year (1981–1982); this increased level in clinical research in the United Kingdom has been maintained in subsequent years[159]. There are several similar examples from other countries. In addition, it is very probable that when regulators themselves conduct a study of their own performance this exercise alone, irrespective of the results obtained, will cause them to rethink their own policies and views.

There is very little reason to think that social and genuine economic interests, if they are properly analysed, will conflict; they may well run parallel. Martin[76] has recently designed an international study of social regulation as a whole to examine the hypothesis that appropriately designed policies can lead to technological responses which are consistent with maintained or improved economic performance. 'From the most optimistic perspective' he remarks 'the promise of that understanding is that it may facilitate the formulation of policy strategies capable of reconciling the goals of workplace, environmental and product safety and quality with the goals of restored growth and employment . . .'

In such work, whether it is limited to the pharmaceutical field or undertaken more generally, the limitations of the objective method have to be recognized. It is very unlikely that one will ever entirely succeed in defining acceptable efficacy, acceptable safety or the acceptable balance between the two in universally applicable terms. As Wardell & Lasagna have pointed out:

> 'Most of the debate between the pharmaceutical industry and the Food and Drug Administration stems from disagreement as to what constitutes evidence of safety and efficacy, whether the available data satisfy the present perceived requirements, whether a particular degree of safety or efficacy is sufficient for the intended use, and what uses should be deemed appropriate. We are deluding ourselves by suggesting that safety and efficacy are adequately or even clearly defined concepts in the present state of the art of clinical pharmacology.'[106]

It must also be recognized that the final result of a scientifically based approach is unlikely to be complete uniformity across the world or even throughout Europe, since the populations of different countries may, as pointed out earlier, genuinely have somewhat different needs. Conclusions drawn from objective studies of limited scope but recklessly applied to all regulation everywhere could result in errors as great as any made in the past; a vital aspect of regulation is that it be adapted to the environment in which it functions. Subject to such reservations, present knowledge indicates that one should proceed to further work which can provide drug regulation with a scientifically more defensible basis than it has usually had in the past. The process of study will have to be a continuous one, for the nature of drug research, production and utilization will continue to develop and may change quite drastically, creating new regulatory problems and needs. The only watchword must be the advancement of the public interest, bearing in mind that that interest is unlikely to be served by an approach which is limited to a narrow view of what the patient – and his doctor – really require.

References

1. Wigmore J.H. (1914): Introduction. In: Hemenway H.B., *Legal Principles of Public Health Administration*. As cited by Curran W.J. and Shapiro E.D. (1970) In: *Law Medicine and Forensic Science*. Little, Brown and Company, Boston and Toronto, at p. 669

2. Penn R.G. (1979): *The state control of medicines: the first 3000 years*. Br. J. Clin. Pharmac., **8**, 293–305

3. Levey, M. (1963): Fourteenth century Muslim medicine and the hisba. *Med. History*, **7**, 176–182

4. Goodall C. (1684): *The Royal College of Physicians of London*. London

5. Dukes M.N.G. (1963): *Patent Medicines and Autotherapy in Society*. Drukkerij Pasmans, The Hague

6. Anon. (1799): On quackery and the most effective means of checking its dangerous progress. *Med. Phys. Journ.*, **1**, 337–340

7. Bruinsma V., Bruinsma G.W. (1878): *De Kwalkalverij met Geneesmiddelen*. Van Belkum Kzn., Leeuwarden

8. United States Senate Documents (1937): **124**, 75th Cong., 2nd sess.

9. Anon. (1969): *Gaps in Technology: Pharmaceuticals*. Report presented to the Third Ministerial Meeting on Science. Organization for Economic Co-operation and Development, Paris

10. Sjöström H. and Nilsdson R. (1972): *Thalidomide and the Power of the Drug Companies*. Penguin Books, Harmondsworth

11. Dunlop, Sir Derrick (1967): The assessment of the safety of drugs and the role of government in their control. *J. Clin. Pharm.*, July–August, 184–192

12. Halse M., Lunde P.K.M. (1978): *Norway* In: Wardell W.M. (ed.) Controlling the use of Therapeutic Drugs. American Enterprise Institute, Washington D.C

13. Fällman H. (1979): 'Vi kan tvingas stoppa nyregistreringarna och koncentrere oss pá befintlinga risker' (interview with Prof. A. Liljestrand). Läkartidningen, **76**, 4767–4769

14. Anon. (1981): *The Control of Drugs for the Elderly*. World Health Organization, Regional Office for Europe, EURO Reports and Studies Nr. **50**, 36pp

15. Anon. (1984): UK data sheets and elderly. *Scrip*, **868**, 5

16. Del Favoro A. (1983): Benoxaprofen. *In*: M.N.G. Dukes (ed.) Side Effects of Drugs Annual, **7**, Excerpta Medica, Amsterdam and Oxford

17. Lundberg G.D. (1983): Why Not Scientific Administration? *J.A.M.A.*, **250**, 2795

18. *HAI News* (1981 onwards): Health Action International, Penang, Malaysia

19. Cook R., Shearer S.B., Strand J. (1982): Contraceptives and Drug Regulation: an International Perspective. *Piact Papers*, **7**, 1–38

20. Anon (1973): *Clinical Pharmacological Evaluation in Drug Control: Proceedings of a Symposium.* W.H.O. Regional Office for Europe

21. Huyghe B. and Torfs-Bruder D. (1979): Harmonization of Registration Procedures for Medicines in Benelux. In: Lahon H., Rondel R.K. and Kratochvil C. (eds.): *Pharmaceutical Medicine – The Future.* Acta Therapeutica. Brussels

22. Dukes M.N.G. (1981): Harmonization of Pharmaceutical Regulation: A Personal View. *Scrip*, **561**, 5–6

23. Wolfe S.M. (1983): *Letter from Health Research Group to the Secretary, Department of Health and Human Services.* Washington, DC, December 28th

24. Cromie B. (1979): Present problems: The effects of British regulations. In: *Medicines for the year 2000.* Office of Health Economics, London

25. James B.G. (1977): *The future of the multinational pharmaceutical industry to 1990.* ABP Ltd. London

26. Idänpään-Heikkilä J. (1983): *A review of safety information obtained from Phases I-II and Phase III Clinical Investigations of sixteen selected drugs.* Department of Health and Human Services, Food and Drug Administration, Rockville MD

27. Marks J., Tayler D. (1983): Measuring the social benefits of medicines. *Pharm. Int.*, **4**, 249–250

28. Jönsson B. (1984): The Social Costs of Adverse Drug Reactions – An Economic View. In: Boström, H. of Ljungstedt, N. (eds.) *Detection and Prevention of Adverse Drug Reactions.* Almqvist & Wiksell, Stockholm

29. Jonsson E. (1974): *Samhällsekonomiska kostnader för vägtraffikolyckor, yrkesskador och rökbetingade sjukdomar.* EFI, Stockholm

30. Bergman U. and Wiholm B.E. (1980): Drug related problems causing admission to a medical clinic. In: Wiholm, B.E–: (ed.): *On the accuracy of drug utilization in health care.* Stockholm

31. Schelling J.L. and Brooke E.M. (1977): *Drug monitoring in hospital.* Lausanne

32. Harcus A.W. (ed.) (1980): *Risk and Regulation in Medicine – the fettered physician.* Association of Medical Advisers in the Pharmaceutical Industry, London

33. Wade O.L. (1980): Instant medicine: A problem of decision making in the glare of publicity. In: Harcus A.W. (ed.): *Risk and Regulation in Medicine.* Association of Medical Advisers in the Pharmaceutical Industry, London

34. Griffin J.P. (1980): The sins of the regulator and the regulated. In: Harcus A.W. (ed.): *Risk and Regulation in Medicine.* Association of Medical Advisers in the Pharmaceutical Industry, London

35. Burrell C. (1980): Drug assessment in uproar. In: Harcus A.W. (ed.): *Risk and Regulation in Medicine.* Association of Medical Advisers in the Pharmaceutical Industry, London

36. Quantock D.C. (1980): The effect of regulation on International drug development. In: Harcus A.W. (ed.): *Risk and Regulation in Medicine.* Association of Medical Advisers in the Pharmaceutical Industry, London

37. U.S. Pure Food and Drug Act (1906); Shirley Amendment (1912)

38. Mitchell S.A., and Link E.A. (eds.) (1976): *Impact of Public Policy on Drug Innovation and Pricing.* The American University, Washington D.C.

39. Cooper J.D. (1970): *Regulation, Economics and Pharmaceutical Innovation.* In: Proceedings of the First Seminar on Economics of Pharmaceutical Innovation, The American University, Washington D.C.

40. Hansen R.W. (1978): *The Impact of Public Policy on Pharmaceutical Innovation.*

Presentation at the American Economics Association Meetings, August 29th
41. Peltzman S. (1973): An Evaluation of Consumer Protection Legislation: The 1962 Drug Amendments. *J. Politic. Econ.*, **81**, fn 13, 1067
42. Baily M.N. (1972): Research and Development Cost and Returns: The U.S. Pharmaceutical Industry. *J. Politic. Econ.*, **80**, 70–85
43. Jadlow Jr. J.M. (1970): *The Economic Effects of the 1962 Drug Amendments*. Thesis, University of Virginia
44. Jondrow J.M. (1972): *A Measure of the Monetary Benefits and Costs of the Regulation of Prescription Drug Effectiveness*. Thesis, University of Wisconsin
45. Wardell W.W., Lasagna L. (1975): *Regulation and Drug Development*. American Enterprise Institute for Public Policy Research. Washington D.C.
46. Grabowski H.G. (1976): *Drug Regulation and Innovation: Empirical Evidence and Policy Options*. American Enterprise Institute for Public Policy Research, Washington D.C.
47. Schwartzman D. (1976): *Innovation in the Pharmaceutical Industry*. Johns Hopkins University Press, Baltimore MD
48. Ashford N.A., Butler S.E., Zolt E.M. (1977): Regulation and Innovation in the Pharmaceutical Industry. Manuscript, 32 pp.
49. Hattis D., Andrews R., Estes J.W., Owen S.T., Ashford N.A. (1980): *Relationships between Aspects of Pharmaceutical Regulation, Innovation and Therapeutic Benefits*. Phase 1, Final Report. Nr. CPA–80–15. Centre for Policy Alternatives, M.I.T., Cambridge, Mass
50. Dukes M.N.G. and Lunde I. (1981): The Regulatory Control of Non-Steroidal Anti-Inflammatory Agents. *Eur. J. Clin. Pharm.*, **19**, 3–10
51. Wieringa N. (1983): *Registratie van Bèta-Blokkers*: Unpublished dissertation, University of Groningen, 97 pp.
52. Haayer F.M., van der Werf G. Th., Wieringa N.F. and Wesseling H. (1983): Use of Cimetidine: Parallels and Discrepancies Between the Views of Drug Regulatory Agencies and Practising Physicians. *Eur. J. Clin. Pharm.*, **25**, 601–7
53. Dukes M.N.G., and Lunde I. (1982): Review of restrictive actions under the Australian drug regulatory system. *Med. J. Austr.*, May 15th, 412–416
54. Hansen R.W. (1976): *Regulation and Pharmaceutical Innovation: A Review of the Literature on Monetary Measures and Costs and Benefits*. Paper prepared for the National Science Foundation
55. Lunde I and Dukes M.N.G. (1981): On Regulating Regulation. *Eur. J. Clin. Pharm.*, **19**, 1–2
56. Steward F., Wibberley G. (1980): Drug innovation – what's slowing it down? *Nature*, **284**, 118–120
57. Dukes M.N.G., Lunde I. (1979): Controls, common sense and communities. *Pharm. Weekbl.*, **114**, 1283–94
58. Griffin J.P. and D'Arcy P.F. (1981): Adverse reactions to drugs – the information lag. In: Dukes M.N.G. (ed.): *Side Effects of Drugs Annual*, **5**, Excerpta Medica, Amsterdam and Oxford
59. Simonian S., van Gessel H. and Beekhof H. (1981): A retrospective analysis of drug carcinogenicity and mutagenicity data. *Pharm. J.*, January 17th, 59–61
60. Heywood R. (in press 1984): *Prediction of Adverse Drug Reactions from Animal Safety Studies*. Paper presented to the Skandia International Symposium on Adverse Reactions, Stockholm, October 1983
61. Griffin J.P., and Diggle G.E. (1981): A Survey of Products Licenced in the United Kingdom from 1971–1981. *Br. J. clin. Pharm.*, **12**, 453–463
62. Zbinden, G. and Flury-Roversi M. (1981): Significance of the LD_{50} test for the toxicological evaluation of chemical substances. *Arch. Toxicol.*, **47**, 77–99

63. Haxthausen S. (1983): *The Right to Know and the Right to Care*. Paper for the WHO Symposium on Clinical Pharmacological Evaluation in Drug Control, Schlangenbad. (Unpublished manuscript)
64. Granat M., Jødal B., Sjöblom T. (1983). The processing of Applications for the Registration of Medicines in the Nordic Countries. *J. Soc. Adm. Pharm.* **1**, 34–44
65. Lunde I., (1984) *The Rejection of New Drugs in Hungary – A Comparative Study*. (Unpublished manuscript)
66. Klaes L., Seebach R., Lex C., Feick J. (1982): *Regulative Politik und politisch-administratve Kultur. En Vergleich von fünf Lädern und vier Interventionsprogrammen*. Unpublished document, Institut für angewandte Sozialforschung, Universität zu Köln.
67. Lunde I. and Dukes M.N.G. (1982): The concept of geriatric drugs: a regulatory dilemma. *Pharm. Int.*, March, 94–98
68. Buurma H., Bodewitz H.J.H.W., Vulto A.G. et al. (1981): De beoordeling van nieuwe geneesmiddelen. *Pharm. Weekbl.*, **116**, 1121–1133
69. Lunde I, Dukes M.N.G. (1980): Les répercussions du contrôle administratif des médicaments: étude comparée de la situation en Norvège et aux Pays-Bas. *Industrie Santé*, **49**, 37–57
70. Offerhaus L. (1984): Novae en andere ongerechtigheden in de farmacotherapie. *Ned. T. Geneesk.*, **128**, 26–30
71. Dukes M.N.G. (1984): *The Registration History of Cromolyn Sodium: a five-country analysis*. (to be published)
72. Grabowski H., Vernon J.M. and Thomas L.G. (1976): The Effects of Regulatory Policy on the Incentives to Innovate: An International Comparative Analysis. In: Mitchell S.A. and Link E.A. (eds.): *Impact of Public Policy on Drug Innovation and Pricing*. The American University, Washington D.C.
73. Wardell W.W. (1976): *Regulation and Pharmaceutical Innovation: A Review of the Relationship Between Government Regulation Aimed at Protecting Health and Human Safety, and Innovation Leading to Medically Useful Drugs*. Unpublished paper
74. Anon. (1983): Leading pharmaceutical companies, 1982–3. *Scrip*, **857–8**, 18–21
75. Anon. (1982): *The Times 1000: Leading companies in Britain and overseas*. Times Books Ltd., London
76. Martin A. (1983): *Social Regulation, Innovation and Technology Policy*. Center for the Study of Policy Alternatives, Boston Mass. (Unpublished manuscript)
77. Young J.H. (1982): Public Policy and Drug Innovation. *Pharmacy in History*, **24**, 1–56
78. Hass A.E., McCormick L.D., Aspel S. *et al* (1982): *A Historical Look at Drug Introductions on a Five-Country Market*. Office of Planning and Evaluation, Food and Drug Administration, Rockville, Md
79. Anon. (1980): *F.D.A. Drug Approval – A Lengthy Process That Delays the Availability of Important New Drugs*. General Accounting Office, Washington D.C. (HRD–80–64)
80. Anon. (1981): *Patent-Term Extension and the Pharmaceutical Industry*. Congress of the United States, Office of Technology Assessment. Washington, D.C
81. Allen T.J., Utterback J.M., Sirbu M.A. *et al.* (1978): Government influence on the process of innovation in Europe and Japan. *Res. Policy*, **7**, 124–149
82. Grabowski H.G., Vernon J.M. and Thomas L.G. (1978): Estimating the effects of regulation on innovation: An international comparative analysis of the Pharmaceutical Industry. *J. Law Commerce*. **21**, 133–63
83. Sune Larsson K., Elwin C.E., Gabrielsson J. *et al.* (1982): Do Teratogenicity Tests serve their Objectives? *Lancet*, **2**, August 21st, 439

84. Personal Communication
85. Wells N. (1983): *Pharmaceutical Innovation: Recent trends, future prospects.* Office of Health Economics, London
86. May M.S., Wardell W.M., Lasagna L. (1983): New drug development during and after a period of regulatory change: Clinical research activity of major United States pharmaceutical firms, 1958 to 1979. *Clin. Pharm. Ther.*, **33**, 691–700
87. Denkewalter R.G., and Tischler M. (1966): Drug Research – Whence and Whither. in: Jucker E. (ed.): *Progress in Drug Research.* Birkhauser, Basel
88. Schmidt A.M. (1977), as cited in *Business Week*, Feb 21st, p.82
89. Foster A. (ed.) (1983): *Drug injury and what to do about it.* Inter-Action Inprint, London
90. Hutt P.B. (1983): Investigations and reports respecting FDA regulation of new drugs. *Clin. Pharm. Ther.*, **33**, 537–548 and 674–687
91. Grabowski H. (1982): Public Policy and Innovation: the Case of Pharmaceuticals. *Technovation*, **1**, 157–189
92. Conversations with R&D Staff of Pharmaceutical Companies during the preparation of the studies 1983–4
93. *Scrip* (1984): Reports on ICI Pharmaceuticals Division (p.6) and Hoffman-La Roche (p.7)
94. Grabowski H.G. and Vernon J.M. (1982): A sensitivity analysis of expected profitability of pharmaceutical R&D. *Managerial and Decision Economics*, **3**
95. Schmidt, A. (1974): *The FDA Today: Critics, Congress and Consumerism.* Speech to National Press Club, Washington, D.C., October 29th. (as cited by Grabowski, reference 91)
96. Culyer A.J. and Horisberger B. (1983): *Economic and Medical Evaluation of Health Care Technologies.* Springer-Verlag, Berlin
97. Weisbrod B.B. (1983): *Economic Approaches to Evaluating a New Medical Technology: The Drug Cimetidine.* In: Culyer and Horisberger (see Ref. 96) at pp. 188–205
98. Horisberger B. (1983): *A Review of the Epidemiological Development of Peptic Ulcers and an Evaluation of Duodenal Ulcers in the Federal Republic of Germany Before and After Cimetidine.* In: Culyer and Horisberger (see Ref. 96) at pp. 213–236
99. Bloom B.S. (1983): *Discussion of Paper by Horisberger.* In: Culyer and Horisberger (see Ref. 96) at pp. 213–236
100. Sonnenberg A., Fritsch A. and Sonnenberg G.S. (1983): *Discussion of Paper by Weisbrod.* In: Culyer and Horisberger (see Ref. 96) at pp. 206–210
101. Jönsson B. (1983): *A Review of the Macroeconomic Evaluation of Cimetidine.* In: Culyer and Horisberger (see Ref. 96) at pp. 243–261
102. Dukes M.N.G. (1973): Role of Data on Comparative Efficacy in Drug Approval. In: *Report of the Second Symposium on the Clinical Pharmacological Evaluation in Drug Control.* World Health Organization, Regional Office for Europe, Copenhagen. EURO 7407
103. Data from Paul de Haen Inc., as quoted in Cooper J.D. (1969): *The Economics of Drug Innovation.* The American University, Washington D.C. at p. 126
104. Gelzer J. (1979): Government toxicology regulations: an encumbrance to drug research? *Arch. Toxicol.* **43**, 19–26
105. Ashford N.A. and Heaton G.R. (1984): Regulation and Technological Innovation in the Chemical Industry. *Law and Contemp. Probl.*, **46**, 501–549
106. Wardell W.W. and Lasagna L. (1975): *Regulation and Drug Development.* American Enterprise Institute for Public Policy Research, Washington D.C.
107. Anon. (1984): Only 14 drugs approved in 1983 in U.S. *Scrip*, 862, 12

108.   Saks D.F. (1979): The Resurgence in New Drug Activity. *Wertheim Industry Commentary*. February 7th, p.8
109.   Anon. (1975): *National Support for Science and Technology: An Explanation of the Foreign Experience*. Center for Policy Alternatives, Boston, Mass. Nr. CPA 75–12/V.2
110.   Crout J.R. (1981): *The Drug Regulatory System: Reflections and Predictions*. Transcript of a speech presented at the Food and Drug Law Institute
111.   Cook J., Prunella P., Stringer S. *et al* (1980): *Approvals and Non-approvals of New Drug Applications during the 1970's*. FDA Bureau of Drugs, Rockville Md. OPE Study 57
112.   Hass A.E. Jr. (1983) *Marketing Patterns of Top-Selling New Drugs in Eleven Countries*. FDA Office of Planning and Evaluation (Unpublished manuscript)
113.   Steward H.F., Wibberley G. (1980): Drug innovation – what's slowing it down? *Nature*, **284**, 118–120
114.   Steward H.F. (1978): Public Policy and Innovation in the Drug Industry. In: Black D. and Thomas G.P. (eds.): *Providing for the Health Services*. Croom Helm, London 1978
115.   Peretz S.M. (1980): *An Industry Viewpoint on Harmonization of National Drug Regulatory Requirements*. Lunchtime Address to FDA/WHO International Conference of Drug Registration Authorities, Annapolis Maryland. (Unpublished Manuscript)
116.   Conzen W.H. (1980): *The Pharmaceutical Industry's Views on International Communication Among Drug Registration Authorities*. Lunchtime Address to the FDA/WHO International Conference of Drug Registration Authorities, Annapolis, Maryland. (Unpublished Manuscript)
117.   Anon. (1980): *Comments and Recommendations on Drug Registration*. International Federation of Pharmaceutical Manufacturers Associations, Zurich
118.   Kristinsdottir G. (1982): *Registration of pharmaceutical specialities in Iceland*. Paper presented to the Second International Conference of Drug Regulatory Authorities, Rome
119.   Loutsch-Weydert (1982): *Registration of Drugs in Luxemburg*. Paper presented to the Second International Conference of Drug Regulatory Authorities, Rome
120.   Hemminki E. (1981): Noninvestigational Use of Unapproved Drugs – Experience from the Scandinavian Countries. *Medical Care*, **19**, 1056–60
121.   Clarren S.N., Nalley P.G., Zuiches C. (1982): *The experiment in Post-Marketing Surveillance of prescription Drugs: An Initial Status Report*. National Bureau of Standards. Washington D.C.
122.   Hartley K., Maynard A. (1982): *The Costs and Benefits of Regulating New Product development in the U.K. Pharmaceutical Industry*. Office of Health Economics, London
123.   Lesser F. (1983): Drugs monitor needs sharper teeth. *New Scientist*, March 17th. 729–732
124.   Anon. (1983): Nur Mut – Ein schwarzes Jahr für die Pharma-Industrie. *Der Spiegel*, **40**, 62–77
125.   Griffiths A. (1981): *Pharmaceuticals in Europe's Health Services: An Economic Review*. Paper presented to the Swedish Social Security Committee
126.   Anon. (1982): 1280 Médicaments moins remboursés dès aujourd'hui. *Quotidien du Médecin*. **12**. Nr. 2825, 1
127.   Anon. (1982): Broker pessimistic over Merck & Co. short term, others disagree. *Pharm. Marketletter*, July 26th, 13
128.   Kilgour A. (1982): Whatever happened to Glaxo's shares? *Lancet*, Oct. 16th, 868
129.   Levy R.I., Sondik E.J. (1982): Large-Scale Clinical Trials: Are they worth the

cost? *Ann. N.Y. Acad. Sci.*, 411–22

130. ten Ham, M. (1983): De toelating van geneesmiddelen in Nederland. *Ned. Tijdschr. Geneesk.*, **127**, 968–71

131. Bristow A.F., Bangham D.R. (1981) The control of medicines produced by recombinant DNA technology. *TIPS*, August, VI–VIII

132. Defoe D. (1722): *A Journal of the Plague Year*. London

133. Bezold C. (ed.) (1983): *Pharmaceuticals in the Year 2000. The Changing Context for Drug R&D*. Institute for Alternative Futures, Alexandra, Va

134. Labour Party (1976): *Discussion document on the Pharmaceutical Industry*. London

135. Anon. (1983): *The Use of Essential Drugs*. World Health Organization, Geneva. Technical Report Series Nr. 685

136. St. George D. and Fraper P. (1981): A Health Policy for Europe. *Lancet*, August 29th 463–465

137. Walker S.R., Scheutz E., Schuppan D., Gelzer J. (1983): *A comparative retrospective analysis of data from short and long-term animal toxicity studies on 40 pharmaceutical compounds*. (Unpublished manuscript)

138. Bruun K. (ed.) (1982): *Läkemedels frógan i Norden*. Bokförlaget Prisma, Stockholm

139. Smith A. (1980): Drug famine: possible solutions. *Brit. Med. J.* **281**, 1475–77

140. Ballin J.C. (1981): Trends in Regulation and Development of New Drugs. *J.A.M.A.*, **245**, 2161–2163

141. Schou J. (1981): Haemmes terapeutiske fremskridt af sikkerhedskravene til laegemidler? *Ugeskr. Laeg.*, **143**, 1670–1672

142. Anon. (1983): Avslåtte registreringssoeknader. *Nytt fra Statens legemiddelkontroll*, **1**, 13

143. Lunde I. and Lunde P.K.M. (1984): The effect of regulatory measures on drug utilization in Norway. (Unpublished draft manuscript)

144. Hadler N.M. (1984): The argument for aspirin as the NSAID of choice in the management of rheumatoid arthritis. *Drug Intell. Clin. Pharm.*, **18**, 34–38

145. Anon. (1984): Confidentiality and the UK CSM. *Scrip*, **859**, 22

146. Anon. (1984): Italian product suspensions. *Scrip*, **862**, 1

147. Anon. (1984): Study criticizes Dr Temple. *Scrip*, **868**, 8

148. Anon. (1984): Consumerists want 'butazones' banned. *Scrip*, **860**, 20

149. Teeling-Smith G. (ed.) (1983): *Measuring the Social Benefits of Medicine*. Office of Health Economics, London

150. Collier J., New L. (1984): Illegibility of Drug Advertisements. *Lancet*, February 11th. 341

152. Cox R.B., Griffin J.P., Allen P.: The free movement of medicines in Europe: a survey. *Pharmacy International* (1983). **4**, 80–82

153. Sancho-Garnier H. (1984): Personal Communication

154. Crout J.R. (1983): Personal Communication

155. Nordisk Lakemedelsstatistik 1978–1980; Nordic Council on Medicines (1982). 135

156. Annual reports of the Committee on Safety of Drugs and subsequently of the Medicines Commission (Committee on Safety of Medicines)

157. Lens J. and Laporte J.R. (1984): Personal Communication

158. Twomey C.E.J., Griffin J.P. (1983), The Information Lag: has it improved. *Pharmacy International*. **4**, 57–61

159. Speirs C.J., Griffin J.P. (1983): A survey of the first year of operation of the new procedure affecting the conduct of clinical trials in the United Kingdom. *Br. J. Clin. Pharmac.* **15**, 649–655

160. Crout J.R. (1983): Personal Communication
161. Ashford, Priest, Hattisd et al: Estimating the benefits of environmental health and safety regulations (1982): MIT Center for Policy Alternatives
162. Bell N. Kûnstige Regelung fûr den freien Verleehr mit Arrneispesialitaten. 1984. Pharm Ind. **46**, 129–134
163. Barker M. Approaching the Millenium. (1983)
164. Ravenscroft M.K. and Walker S.R. (1984). Innovation as assessed by new chemical entities marketed in the United Kingdom between 1960 and 1982. British Journal of Pharmacology (in press)
165. Dayan A. (1981): The relative work of animal testing. Risk-benefit analysis – Drug Research. (ed). Cavalla J.P. pp 97–112. M.T.P. Press Lancaster
166. Walker S.R. (1982): Innovation and drug development – can the process be expedited? Bira Journal. 34–42
167. Lumley C.E. and Walker S.R. (1984): The establishment of a computer-based toxicology databank. Presentation at the British Toxicology Society Meeting (March 1984)
168. Griffin J.P. (1984): Contribution to the discussion, W.H.O. Meeting on the European Studies of Drug Regulation, Oslo, March 1984
169. Laporte J.R. (1984): Contribution to the discussion, W.H.O. Meeting on the European Studies of Drug Regulation, Oslo, March 1984
170. Fatturusso V. (1979): Relations between the community regulations and WHO technical activity in the drug sector: In Poggiolini D., (ed.): The future of the EEC procedures for the harmonization of drug registration. Academic Press, London
171. Anon. (1984): Aleotti on 'death' of Italian industry. Scrip, **905**, 1
172. Dukes M.N.G. (1984): The Seven Pillars of Foolishness. In Dukes M.N.G. (ed.) Side Effects of Drugs Annual, **8**, Elsevier, Amsterdam and Oxford
173. Crout J.R. (1984): Contribution to the discussion, W.H.O. Meeting on the European Studies of Drug Regulation, Oslo, March 1984
174. Kennedy D. (1984): In whose best interest? The Stanford Magazine, **12**, Nr. 2 50–56
175. Berlin H., Jönsson B. (1984): Livslängd, Aelder, Förnyelse. Liber Forlag, Malmö
176   McNamara B.P. (1976): Long term versus short term toxicity tests. In: Mehlman M.A. et al. (eds.) Concepts in Health Evaluation of Commercial and Industrial Chemicals. Wiley, New York

Annex 1

LIST OF PARTICIPANTS

Ms Solveig Andersen
Norwegian Medicines Control
    Authority
Sven Oftedals vei 6
Oslo 9
Norway

Dr N. Ashford
Director
Center for Policy Alternatives
Massachusetts Institute of
    Technology
Cambridge, Massachusetts 02139
USA

Professor Istvan Bayer
Director-General
National Institute of Pharmacy
PO Box 450
H-1372 Budapest 5
Hungary

Professor N.H. Choulis
Dean, School of Pharmacy
University of Athens
104 Solonos Street
Athens 144
Greece

Dr J. Richard Crout
Director, Office of Medical
    Applications of Research
National Institutes of Health
Building 1, Room 216
Bethesda, MD 20205
USA

Dr J.P. Griffin
Professional Head of Medicines
    Division
Department of Health and Social
    Security
Committee on Safety of Medicines
Market Towers
1 Nine Elms Lane
London SW8 5NQ
United Kingdom

Mr Almar Grimsson
Chief, International Health Affairs
Ministry for Health and Social
    Security
(Heilbrigdis og
    Tryggingamalaraduneytid)
Laugavegur 116
IS-105 Reykjavik
Iceland

Professor M. Hassar
Professeur de pharmacologie
   clinique
Hôpital Avicenne
Rabat
Morocco

Dr J. Idänpään-Heikkilä
Chief Medical Officer for
   Pharmacology
The National Board of Health
Siltasaarenkatu 18 A
SF-00530 Helsinki 53
Finland

Mr O. Jennane
Secretaire général du Ministère de la
   Santé publique
335, avenue Mohammed V
Rabat
Morocco

Mr B. Jøldal
Director, Pharmaceutical
   Department
The Health Services of Norway
PO Box 8128 Dep.
N-Oslo 1
Norway

Dr J.-R. Laporte
Divisio de Farmacologia Clinica
Universitat Autonoma de Barcelona
P. Vall d'Hebron s.n.
Barcelona 32/35
Spain

Dr Carlos Lens
Instituto Nacional de la Salud
Servicio de Prestaciones
   Farmaceuticas
Alcala 56
Madrid
Spain

Professor P.K.M. Lunde
Chairman
Department of
   Pharmacotherapeutics
University of Oslo
PO Box 1065 Blindern
Oslo 3
Norway

Dr T. Mork
Director-General
The Health Services of Norway
PO Box 8128 Dep.
N-Oslo 1
Norway

Mr K. Øydvin
WHO Collaborating Centre for
   Drug Statistics Methodology
Norsk Medisinal Depot
Sven Oftedals vei 10
Oslo 9
Norway

Dr James Parker
Vice-President
Fisons Corporation
Two Preston Court
Bedford, Mass 01730
USA

Dr Hélène Sancho-Garnier
Chef de Service
Institut Gustave Roussy
Rue Camille Desmoulins
94805 Villejuif Cedex
France

Dr David Sharp
Assistant Editor
The Lancet
7 Adam Street
London WC2 6AD
United Kingdom

Dr Tony Smith
Assistant Editor
British Medical Journal
British Medical Association
Tavistock Square
London WC1H 9JR
United Kingdom
(Editorial Secretary)

Professor Kjell Strandberg
Director, Bureau of Drugs
National Board of Health and
    Welfare
Department of Drugs
Box 607
S-751 25 Uppsala
Sweden

Dr C.A. Tiejgeler
Chairman
College ter beoordeling van
    geneesmiddelen
(Board for the Evaluation of
    Medicines)
PO Box 439
2260 AK Leidschendam
Netherlands

Dr Stuart Walker
Director
Centre for Medicines Research
Woodmansterne Road
Carshalton
Surrey SM5 4DS
United Kingdom

Professor L. Werkö
AB Astra
S-151 85 Södertalje
Sweden

Mr W.A. Baker (*Editorial Secretary*)
Imperial Chemical Industries (ICI)
Pharmaceuticals Division
Mereside Alderley Park
Macclesfield
Cheshire SK10 4TG
United Kingdom

Ms Marianne Granat
Secretary-General
Nordic Council on Medicines
PO Box 607
S-751 25 Uppsala
Sweden

Mr A. Trostheim
Administrative Director
Norsk Medisinal Depot
Sven Oftedals vei 10
Oslo 9
Norway

WORLD HEALTH ORGANIZATION

Regional Office for Europe
Dr M.N.G. Dukes, Regional Officer for Pharmaceuticals and Drug
Utilization
Ms Geneviève Pinet, Regional Officer for Health Legislation
Inga Lunde, Consultant, Pharmaceuticals and Drug Utilization

Headquarters
Dr M. ten Ham, Pharmaceuticals Unit

Index